ELDERWOMAN

Reap the wisdom... feel the power... embrace the joy

Marian Van Eyk McCain

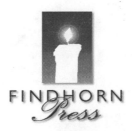

FINDHORN
Press

© Marian Van Eyk McCain 2002

First published by Findhorn Press 2002

ISBN 1 899171 29 0

British Library Cataloguing-in-Publication Data.
A catalogue record for this book is available from
the British Library.

Edited by Lynn Barton
Cover Illustration © Brian Nobbs 2002
Cover design by Thierry Bogliolo
Layout by Pam Bochel

Printed and bound by WS Bookwell, Finland

Published by
Findhorn Press
305a The Park, Findhorn
Forres IV36 3TE
Scotland, UK

tel 01309 690582
fax 01309 690036
e-mail: info@findhornpress.com

findhornpress.com

For two elderwomen of the past, in loving memory:

Susan Manicom, my grandmother,
and Mary Worley, my mother.

And for two elderwomen of the future, with my blessings:

Mia Anderson and Astrid Manfield Mackenzie,
my beloved daughters.

Table of Contents

INTRODUCTION

As a little girl, I longed for curly hair.

Every now and then, if I badgered her enough, Grandma would agree to twist my hair up in rags at bedtime. As she wound the strands of my brown, straight hair up tightly with those strips of cloth, I would sometimes yelp, for it was a rather painful process. "Pride must pinch," she would say sagely, as she went on winding.

It would be an uncomfortable night. But next morning, for a glorious hour after the rags came out, I would have a head full of tumbling ringlets. It was worth the pain, and the wait, to look in the mirror at those swirling curls.

By lunchtime, of course, nothing would be left of all that glory save the faint trace of a wave. And by bedtime my brown tresses would be straight once again. Straight, Grandma would have said, as a yard of pump water.

But I kept trying.

"Am I pretty?" I would ask, longing to be told that I was.

"Only when you smile," would come the answer.

I smile to myself now, as I look at my (still straight) gray hair in the bathroom mirror and think back. Back to the confused and emotional woman in her fifties, struggling to understand the menopause process. Back to the efficient, capable career woman in her forties, and beyond her to the young mother in her thirties, baking her own bread and telling bedtime stories to her daughters. Before that, to the young woman in her sexually charged twenties on her quest for identity, longing for glamour and excitement. Before that to the confused and embarrassed teenager. And before her, to that little girl who so badly wanted to be pretty and have curly hair that she suffered all the discomfort of sleeping with her hair in rags.

It is as though they are different people. So different, in fact, that I can hardly believe they really were all just different versions of me at various stages.

I suppose that to others I have always looked much the same. Just as others look the same to me, year after year, except for the gradual changes which come with aging.

The other day, I came across my mother's wedding photographs and was struck once again by the fact that both my grandmothers, although they were only in their early fifties then, already looked surprisingly old. It was not that their faces were lined, but more that they dressed like old women. Matrons—now there is a good word. Yes, they looked matronly.

Today's fifty-year-olds rarely look matronly. Today's fifty-year-olds are a new breed altogether. And today's forty-year-olds and thirty-year-olds will be looking to their older sisters to show them how to do this aging thing which we all have to do, but which they will want to do in a conscious, empowered way that suits the new millennium.

I had no one to show me that. I tried to figure it out for myself as I went along. I had a wonderful role model in the form of my own grandmother, but although I valued her ways tremendously, I knew they would need adapting if they were to be suitable for me, and for this modern era.

Grandma was a hard-working woman, who lived a simple life, with few material possessions and little stress. She was brimful of wisdom, and dispensed it gently and subtly, without preaching. Her spiritual beliefs were strong and certain, her morality impeccable. She hummed as she went about her daily tasks. She always appeared relaxed and contented, and her face usually wore a smile. She walked everywhere, or caught a bus. She re-used, repaired, recycled and improvised. In many ways, the life she lived would have fit perfectly with these days of increased ecological awareness. But she belonged to her own times, as I belong to mine.

So I decided that if she was to be a role model of sorts for my own old age, then my challenge would have to be to bring all the simple values and pleasures of her life forward into today's scene and adapt them into a form which is suitable for the twenty-first century, for me, and for others like myself who seek to make a difference in the world. That seemed like a big challenge, for the world has changed a lot since she last lived in it.

My grandmother was lucky in some ways. She was not subjected to the enormous conform-or-perish pressures of the consumer society, the tyranny of advertising or the dominance of the youth culture, all of which make aging a more difficult process for women today. Neither was she analytical or introspective. She was, in fact, a simple peasant woman. So aging, for her, was a straightforward, angst-free process which she accepted with little thought. For her modern counterpart, it is often more problematical.

My grandmother taught me how to grow vegetables, but she could not foresee the tragic loss of heritage seed varieties by modern developments in agriculture, horticulture and genetic engineering. She taught me to cook, but she knew nothing about the problems caused by unhealthy diets or the effects of supermarkets upon the High Street economy. She taught me to sew, but she was unaware of the exploitation of workers in offshore sweatshops, and the problems of pesticide use on cotton crops.

She fed the birds in her garden, yet had no idea how much those bird numbers would decline over the next fifty years. Neither would she have realized, as she looked around the full pews in her church on Sunday, that the world around her was entering an era of severe spiritual crisis. Her horizons were confined to her family, her church, and her neighborhood. She listened to the radio, but never owned a TV and probably never heard the word "computer" in her life. Her siblings and friends were much like her.

I always hoped that I would be a lot like her too, in my own old age, but I also knew that for me there had to be something more, something of which she would have known little, at least in a conscious way. This book, as well as being a tribute to her, is an investigation into that "something more."

For me, one of the best ways to figure something out is to write it down. This book you are now reading is the second installment of my writing on the subject of aging. The first was a book about menopause.[1] So for the benefit of those who have not read that first installment, I will briefly review the whole topic of menopause in Chapter 2. This is an important topic because menopause is the doorway into the third age of womanhood. I believe that the way we "do" menopause determines, to a great extent, how ready we are going to be to accept the challenges of old age.

The latter part of our lives, as Carl Jung pointed out so eloquently, is meant to be lived according to a different rhythm. Yet there is scant teaching in our society, as yet, on how this should be done. As he put it:

*Thoroughly unprepared we take the step into the
afternoon of life; worse still, we take this step with the
false assumption the our truths and ideals will serve us as
hitherto. But we cannot live the afternoon of life
according to the program of life's morning… How many
of us older ones [are] really prepared for the second half
of life, for old age, death and eternity?… The afternoon
of life must also have a significance of its own and cannot
be merely a pitiful appendage to life's morning.*[2]

This book is my attempt to sketch out some notes about what I see as my own program for the "afternoon of life." It is a map my own fifty-year-old self would have welcomed, a map my forty-year-old, or even thirty-year-old self might have looked forward to peeking at. Since I found no pre-existing maps available—just a few fragments here and there—more like scribbled notes on the backs of envelopes than proper maps—I had to create my own. Having begun to create it, I find that it remains a "work in progress." Nevertheless, I hope this working copy may be useful to others. It is more than I had, at any rate.

Lately, I have asked a number of women younger than myself what kind of map they would like to guide them into their own third age. I have asked them what their fears are. What their concerns are. How they imagine it will be for them. Many of the young ones, in their thirties and forties, say that they cannot even begin to imagine it. They cannot see around the bend of menopause. And yet they are curious, already, to know what is really there. And they are determined that it will not be an empty space, although they are fearful that it could be. They sense and hope that in so-called 'retirement' they will remain involved with the world in ways that are larger than the simple tasks of grandparenting or tending their gardens. They sense that there will be a lightening and they are curious to know what forms it will take. They sense that they will have more permission to express their true feelings and personalities in the world, and they grin with delight at the thought of how outrageous they might allow themselves to be when they are old women. How crabby and persnickety and obstinate they might decide to be. They already know that they will "wear purple…and learn to spit." And, to my surprise, despite the popular criteria of beauty which pervade our youth-obsessed culture, their poetry contains wonderful images of the special beauty of the old woman's body.

> *...around her secateurs the curling hand*
> *is like a polished vine, and her bare legs*
> *the narrow trunks of birches, for a while*
> *she has been turning tree-like.*[3]

I really do believe that the coming generations, unlike my mother's and my own, are going to march into old age with their sense of inner power intact and not submit to being discounted, forgotten and ignored and relegated to a life of bingo and TV interspersed with trips to the mall. So there is a huge energy resource there. I believe that it is potentially one of the biggest and most important resources for social change, and I am meeting increasing numbers of people who share this view. It is an exciting prospect.

It seems to me that the increasing lightness of old age lends itself perfectly to a conscious divesting of "stuff" and a deepening understanding of the meaning of "living lightly on the Earth." Even in the elderly folk I have known whose level of political awareness is not particularly high, I see a natural tendency to lighten their ballast, give things away, eat less, need a smaller range of clothes as they age, and so on. And in the ones whose social and environmental consciousness is high, there is a corresponding change in their reference point; a tendency to identify with wider issues and realities beyond the personal. The philosopher Bertrand Russell, in his nineties, spoke of spreading himself more thinly over a wider and wider area as he aged, and I meet many women who express a sense of that same spreading-out process. Like Florida Scott-Maxwell, who wrote, in her eighties, about her great surprise at finding herself caring more and more passionately about issues than she had in her earlier life, even though the energy to act out of that passion had to be more carefully husbanded,[4] we meet more and more elders who remain fully involved with the wider concerns of their societies and of the planet itself.

So if you put together the large group of empowered individuals due to come on the scene over the next few decades, the developmental experience of post-menopausal "lightening" and the heightened contemporary interest in social and environmental issues, you have a potential company of gray-haired women whose combined energy is phenomenal. What a resource to harness! Not that every older woman in years to come will be out there marching in demonstrations. Far from it. The grandmothering phase of life is a phase of gentle, subtle influence, often wielded at a very local level, within a small group of family and friends or a local community. The point I am trying to make is not that tomorrow's grandmothers will be Amazons, but that they will be women whose global vision informs their lives in a way that my own grandmother's never did. Women who grow old with the Internet will never be content to believe that the world ends at their kitchen walls, even if their physical mobility is one day tied to a Zimmer frame.

But those menopausal years form a bend in the path. From forty, you cannot possibly see through to what sixty-five might feel like, let alone eighty-five. Therefore, although I know from personal experience, and from contact with a number of post-menopausal women who feel as I do, that I am on to something, it may be hard to explain this in a convincing way to someone who has not yet felt the first stirrings of it. That, for me, is the challenge of writing this book. I want to bring to every woman who fears the loss of her youth, the wrinkling of her skin or the waning of her sex appeal, the promise of new riches to come and the new sense of purpose which can be hers in this fruitful time of life we call the third age.

If you flip idly through pages that follow, you will notice many things which may surprise you. The stages of womanhood, well yes, that is a good starting point; menopause, yes, that is relevant. But what, you may wonder, does the composition of soil have to do with getting old? Why this whole section on animals? Goddesses, well maybe, but why on Earth is this crazy woman going on about such seemingly irrelevant things as Santa Claus, snakes, bungee jumping, airplane journeys and compost heaps?

Well it will make sense, as you read it, I promise. Because this is not simply a book about growing old. It is a book about growing up and out and in and down and into. It invites you to grow up to your fullest possible height—metaphorically speaking—and to grow out into the world in a whole new way. It challenges you to grow in—into the deep and rich and fascinating inner life of your soul, and down into a new relationship with the Earth. And it invites you to grow into a new type of person. A wiser, deeper, more joyful person than you ever thought you could be. An old age consciously, fully and deeply lived is a luxury most of our foremothers never had. It is only in our own times that so many women can look forward to another three decades or more of satisfying life post-menopause, which is one of the reasons why there are so few maps for us to follow and an excellent reason for starting to create them now.

So first, I shall be presenting an overview of the stages of our female lives, followed by some details of the menopause process. Then we shall begin to consider what it is that makes the essential difference between being an old woman and being an elderwoman. Using the framework of the Greek elements—earth, air, fire and water—we shall go on to examine this in more detail. As we go, we shall dissect out the principles upon which the elderwoman's life is based.

Like any other old woman, I like to tell my stories. Telling each other our stories is a traditional way that women have always shared their knowledge and their wisdom. And as you read my stories and my ideas on who and what the elderwoman is, I hope that you will bring forward your own ideas and stories also. Maybe you will write some of them down in your journal, if you keep one. Or if you don't keep one, maybe this is a good time to start. I hope you will take time, as you read, to imagine your own part in our dialogue, as though we were sitting together around the fire, passing the talking stick around our circle. Reflect on your own experience. Try out the exercises I have suggested along the way. Think back to your own procession of different selves, from the you of today all the way back to the little girl you once were.

It is a long time now, since I prayed for curly hair. So long, that the memory is fading, like an old snapshot. It is as though I were now looking through a window at that child who yearned for ringlets. I can no longer get inside her mind.

In the same way, the griefs and losses and stresses of menopause, although they seem big at the time, really do fade. If you are willing to take the courageous step of embracing the aging process instead of fighting it, there comes a point at which you laugh at the thought that it ever mattered whether or not anyone called you pretty.

Not only have I got used to the fact that no one wolf-whistles at me now, I would actually be disconcerted if they did. My entire definition of beauty has changed. My inside matches my outside, now, in a way I had never expected, and there is a glorious freedom in that. A freedom which has been as well worth the struggle as those long-ago ringlets but which, unlike them, will never disappear.

> *And we will ruffle the grasses with our talk*
> *turning our trunks to the sun*
> *feeling our nipples scrunch in the wind like walnuts.*
> *And who would dare to tell the tree*
> *that she's not beautiful*
> *because she's old.* [5]

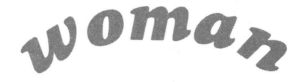

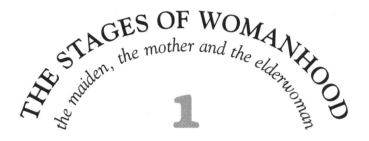

THE STAGES OF WOMANHOOD
the maiden, the mother and the elderwoman
1

CLASSICALLY, a woman's life is divided into three stages. The first is the stage of the maiden, or virgin; the second of the mother; and the third of the crone, or old woman.

This notion of female trinity has been with us since time immemorial, symbolically represented by forms of the goddess. Under many names, such as Hebe-Hera-Hecate in ancient Greece, Juventas-Juno-Minerva in pre-Roman Italy or Mary, Queen of Heaven; Mary, Queen of Earth; and Mary Queen of Hell in Renaissance Europe, the triune, maiden-mother-crone goddess appears throughout history in hundreds of cultures around the world.[1]

In many cultures and mythologies, the stages are equated with the phases of the moon. The new and waxing moon, the full moon, the waning and dark moon all symbolize stages in the waxing and waning of female fertility and, by literal as well as symbolic association, the fertility of the Earth.[2] Although there are few people today, in our Western culture, who perform rituals to the moon goddess, many modern gardeners are fully aware that things planted or transplanted during the waxing moon generally fare better than those planted during its waning phase, and make a point of planting by the moon calendar.

In some tribal cultures, life stages are sharply delineated. The beginning of fertility, particularly, is often marked by ritual. In modern Western culture, this is certainly not the case. Our culture places its emphasis on individual development rather than on rigid and long-established tribal customs. So for us, the stages of a woman's life, although they follow each other sequentially, are less a matter of chronological age and more a matter of our primary relationship with the world. A seventeen-year-old wife with a toddler of her own, for example, may still to all intents and purposes be in the maiden (identity-formation) stage of her emotional development, even though she has physically given birth, while a forty-year-old office manager may be childless and single but be operating very much out of the mother phase, since her identity is well-formed and many of her daily tasks are "generative" ones; in other words, they have to do with creating new things or maintaining existing ones and with the guidance, teaching, discipline and encouragement of other people.

The third member of the female trinity is sometimes referred to as the crone. For many women today, whose minds have been bombarded, since they were little girls, with the propaganda of the beauty industry, the word crone conjures up the image of the wrinkled, warty witch of fairy tales, like the one who tried to eat Hansel and Gretel. Crone derives from the ancient word, "croonie," once used to describe an old ewe who was destined soon to become a meal for crows. It is related to the word "carrion." Not a good look, really.

So I can understand why this word is shocking and repulsive to many women. At the same time, I know that there are increasing numbers who are turning to it and embracing it, precisely because it is such a powerful word. To them it signifies permission to own their increasing sense of personal power, to explore their freedom to be different, to be outrageous, and to experiment with all the hitherto unlived aspects of their own natures.

Women are gathering together, these days, to hold croning ceremonies for their sisters who have reached the menopausal bridge and are crossing over into the third age of their lives (not just in California, either). Since our society has no formal ceremonies for this rite of passage, no way of honoring the shift from the second to the third age of womanhood, it feels good to create one. In this way we mirror, in the outside world, the important inner change which has taken place with the cessation of our bleeding. When my first book, *Transformation Through Menopause*, was published, my women friends used the book launch to create a croning ritual for me as part of the proceedings of the day, and it did, indeed, feel

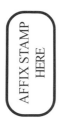

DEEP BOOKS LTD
UNIT 3 GOOSE GREEN TRADING ESTATE
47 EAST DULWICH ROAD
LONDON
SE22 9BN
UK

Thank you for buying this book. If you would like to receive any further information about our product list, please return this card after filling in your areas of interest.

Title of this book..

If purchased : Retailer's name.................................... Town.....................

☐ Health and Nutrition   ☐ Philosophy & Spirituality
☐ Indigenous Cultures   ☐ Psychology & Psychotherapy
☐ Occult & Divination   ☐ Women's Interest
☐ Personal Growth   ☐ Other

Name..
Address...
....

like a very significant moment. We acted out, in word, symbol and song, the three stages of womanhood and honored my passing from the second into the third. And I wore my new crone label with pride.

At the time, I was aware only of the private and personal significance, to me and to other women—my friends, my clients, and the readers of my book—of stepping over the threshold into a new life stage. Although I had explored, in my reading and research, the whole issue of women's power, and taught myself and others to start opening, with courage, to the awesome fullness of it, I had not yet thought deeply into what daily life as a crone might entail. Neither had I grasped the potential social impact of a whole generation of conscious crones upon the world in which I lived. That dawned on me slowly over the years that followed. To my delight, I found that others were having similar thoughts.

Although women are turning with relish to this word "crone" in ever increasing numbers, there are still many for whom it is a distasteful—as it is for the mainstream culture in general. It is only a few hundred years, after all, since the mainstream culture of our forefathers (and I use that word advisedly) ceased to single out its crones for a death sentence. It is estimated that some nine million innocent women were burned as witches—half as many people again as were destroyed by the Holocaust. Even this could well be an underestimate.[3] The echoes of this cruel and tragic slaughter are still with us. It has taken a long time for women to start re-owning their power and coming out as crones. This is hardly surprising. Any species which has been on the verge of extinction takes time to return, especially if the extinction was a deliberate cull, spread over five centuries. The trauma is still detectable in our collective feminine unconscious, just as the dark energies of the Holocaust are still palpable around the precincts of Auschwitz. I have heard many women describe sudden, surprising eruptions of rage and grief deeper than the circumstances of their own lives could ever warrant. Such eruptions are frequently triggered by some relatively minor instance of male oppression and are way out of proportion to the situation. Another common experience, which I believe is related, is an unexpected and unexplained apprehensiveness and blanking out which may arise, apparently from nowhere, when a woman has the impulse to engage in a healing act or is asked by someone for wise counsel. Women who have trained in various healing modalities often experience this sudden uprush of crippling, inexplicable fear when the time comes to hang out the shingle and advertise themselves. When these experiences happen, the women know intuitively that they are tapping into the collective store. I have experienced these strange things myself and been left in no doubt as to where they came from. Unlike my friend Parvati, who believes very literally in past lives and claims to recall, in vivid detail, the scene of her own burning, I make no such assertions. I only know, intuitively, that such feelings come from a far deeper source than my personal self.

However, if we look at why this widespread attack on women happened in the first place, we can see that it was female power—and men's fear of it—which caused such a brutal and massive reaction. For women are powerful, and everyone knows it, instinctively. It is the woman who gives birth and upon whom every human life utterly depends, from the moment of conception to the time of weaning, and usually way beyond. So the awareness of woman as holder of the keys to life and death is built into everyone, male and female alike. While this feels good and natural to most girls and women, in the psyche of the male it can create an ambivalence, love vying with hate, as his need for closeness and dependency clashes with his innate desire for freedom, autonomy and separation.

So there is a sense in which Western society, shaped as it largely is by the psychology of the male, both loves and fears female power. And it seems to me that since she has important work to do over the next phase of human history, we need a word for the powerful old woman in our society which commands instant respect, rather than one—like "crone"— which we have to work long and tediously hard to re-interpret. We cannot spend years convincing men and women alike to look the crone image in the face. They will come to it eventually, but meanwhile, we need another word; one that nobody has to struggle to accept. We need a word with which women will immediately seek to identify and which will remind men that we are a force to be respected—which is why I chose the term "elderwoman."

Not every old woman is an elderwoman, however. Becoming an elderwoman presupposes that we have spent some of our time already on personal development of one kind or another and are continuing to grow in awareness. It assumes that we have become to some degree conscious and aware of ourselves and our inner processes and of the impact our lives have upon the wider world. There is much more to being an elderwoman than simply growing old. And I shall be expanding on this in the chapters which follow.

The triune aspect of femaleness is often expressed as a triangle. The triangle, as we know, is a universal symbol for the female. It echoes the shape of the pubis and represents the three aspects of the goddess holding hands, each aspect being intimately linked with both of the others.

The mother is the link which joins the maiden to the crone. Her body has been the young, flat body of the child and will one day be the old, flat body of the crone. Meanwhile, in her curves, her bleeding and her wetness she speaks to one of what will be and to the other of what has been—and of what has been learned. The crone, being the only one of the three to come into close intimacy with death, gives courage to the mother. Like any other grandmother, she has a special relationship with the youngest— the maiden. In their hand-holding is the delight in play and simple pleasures which is shared by the oldest and the youngest alike. As the crone passes through the portal of death, she brings the promise of new life. For without death there can be no life. So the maiden arises in her place, just as the new apple tree arises from the ground where the apple core was thrown.

Woman, in all her aspects, symbolizes the cyclic nature of all life. In this cycle of eternal renewal, the full and successful completion of each stage is vital to the arising of the next. A girl who does not complete all the developmental tasks of her childhood is ill prepared for the onset of motherhood; a women who cannot let go of her role and face her empty nest comes limping, fearful and reluctant into elderhood; the old woman who remains just an old woman and cannot assume the full mantle of the elderwoman cannot play her vital part in preparing the ground for next year's healthy crop.

One of my grandmother's sayings was that favourite old cliche "If a thing's worth doing, it's worth doing well."

Well, so is being old.

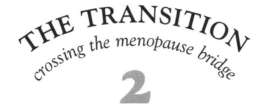

THE TRANSITION
crossing the menopause bridge
2

A FRIEND now in her forties recently wrote this to me:

> I find myself spending extended moments wondering about
> how I will be when I am older. What I need to shed, and
> what I need to keep and what things and parts of me will
> just simply fall away as a necessary part of the process. For
> hints to this I watch my friends, like you and others. I
> watch what they choose to lose and keep and the things
> they lose regardless and the grief they share with me. And I
> add that to my little list of things I can expect and
> sometimes I contemplate how I can prepare myself.
>
> Because my mother was so private and secretive about all
> these things, the process is really self-taught for me. I am
> sure that there will be many women who are like me...
> But the children of women my age, and the many children
> of the women of your age, will have a map of sorts. One
> that they will need to refine, but certainly a clearer one
> than I have had. I am sure there are many who need an
> explorer's map for them to fill in as they might. A few
> beacons to protect against night reefs.

What she may discover, of course, as she heads further into this
transitional phase of her life we call menopause, is that while we are in it,

that time is often very chaotic, confusing and turbulent. Yes, we may have a map of the "night reefs" but that does not necessarily mean that in the dark and fog of our own process we shall not run aground on them over and over again before we are through.

It is like taking a canoe down the rapids. You can study maps of the river, talk to people who have gone that way before, get a sense of where the currents are and the big rocks, and the way a canoe might behave in each circumstance, and have, before you set off, a good idea of what to expect. You may have run those rapids many times in your imagination, or watched videos of someone else negotiating that same stretch of river on a similar sort of day at a similar time of year. But once you are launched, and the current surges under your frail craft, and you feel the power of the river, all other choices are gone. It is just you and the river, then. With the roar of the rapids in your ears, the spray in your face and the powerful surging beneath you, the experience is uniquely your own. It is not the experience of your imagination, nor is it the experience of the person in the video. It is yours, and it is now. You are so busy living it that sometimes it is impossible to understand it completely. Perhaps only later will you be fully able to describe your adventure and to recognize the lessons it taught you.

Luckily, unlike the fast canoe trip, menopause is a slow, gradual process, and despite the typical feelings of chaos and confusion there are occasional periods of clarity within it. There are moments when the fog lifts for a while; times when we can step aside and consider what is going on, making sense of events and feelings which have puzzled or disturbed us.

Let us take a closer look, now, at this menopause process.

Whether she is partnered or single, whether she has followed a career, raised children, traveled the world or stayed home, no matter who she has been in her twenties, thirties and forties, there comes a point in every woman's life when the regular hormonal cycle to which she has become so accustomed begins to wobble and change.

It is as though she learned to ride a bicycle when she was twelve or thirteen, and has become so used to riding everywhere that she has almost forgotten what it was like to walk. There she is, riding merrily along on her bicycle, looking at the scenery, and all of a sudden, she rounds a corner and up ahead is a bridge, a rather narrow, rickety bridge, unsuitable for wheels. So the bicycle slows down and wobbles a little as she gets to the bridge and dismounts. From here, she is going to have to proceed on foot. This is the menopause bridge. The bridge will take her over into the third age of her womanhood, where all her wisdom starts to be harvested.

There is an ancient belief that women's menstrual blood, when it is no longer needed to form babies, turns into wisdom, and that is why older women do not bleed. I love that theory much more than modern medical stories about estrogen.

When I first approached that bridge myself, in the early 1980s, there was very little written about the psychological and spiritual aspects of the so-called change of life. The prevailing attitude among the women of my own generation and the one preceding it was very matter-of-fact. "Just get on with it," they said. "It's nothing to make a fuss about." They pretended it was not happening, or that it was simply a physical thing, an inconvenient stage best hurried through as unobtrusively as possible.

As I began researching menopause, I discovered that the main emphasis, in writing and discussion, was always on the physical aspects— hot flashes, night sweats, etc.—and that the medical profession had deemed it a medical condition rather than a natural life stage. Since medical conditions demand treatment, hormone replacement therapy, with its promises of prolonged youthfulness and of freedom from uncomfortable symptoms, was being aggressively marketed to aging women. This seemed to me problematical, since there was known to be a downside for this treatment, including an increased predisposition to certain types of cancer.

However, there were many women—and I was one of them—who wanted to be fully conscious of the whole process rather than having it medicated away with artificial hormones. We wanted to feel the strange surges of heat—and the buzz that went with them. We wanted to explore our own weird moods and see what hidden doorways of the unconscious mind they revealed. We wanted to meet each challenge as it came and use it for our own growth. We wanted to have the whole adventure— emotional, psychological and spiritual, as well as physical—even if parts of it proved difficult or painful.

I have never regretted that decision, any more than I had regretted the decision to opt for natural childbirth. I do not judge others for not making the same decision, but I am glad that I did it my way. To be sure, there were some rough times. And the whole menopause process, from start to finish, took four or five years to complete. But it was one of the greatest learning times of my whole life.

During my research I found, to my surprise, that the menopausal phase begins, for many women, several years in advance of any physical signs. It is often heralded by certain types of dreams.[1] Dreams about dying mothers are common, as are dreams about neglected or forgotten babies. It is as though the psyche is letting go of its strong identification with the mothering role. This seems to happen to women who have never been biological or adoptive mothers just as much as to those who have. Whether or not they have included childbearing and child-rearing, most women's lives, during those mature years, have incorporated the mothering role in some form. Between our mid-twenties and our mid-fifties, most of us are expressing our creativity and our productiveness in one way or another, whether or not that literally involves children. To birth a project, guide a student, take responsibility for something outside of ourselves—all these are a kind of motherhood. Menopause signals the beginning of the transition from the mothering phase of our lives to the grandmothering phase. (Once again, this does not depend on literally having grandchildren.) And the tasks of the grandmothering phase are, in many ways, quite different, although the difference may not be immediately apparent.

Menopause brings mental and emotional changes, often noticeable some time before the physical ones start to manifest. A certain foggy-mindedness, of the kind we formerly associated with being pre-menstrual, becomes increasingly pervasive. Feelings start to become sharper and moods more volatile. We may become more than usually forgetful.

Menopause is not only a big transition; it is a collection of little transitions too. It is as though we are given a folder full of tasks and we have to complete each one. They can be done in any order, but all must be completed before we can graduate. Some tasks will be easier than others, depending on the individual.

Coming to terms with the end of fertility is a big task for some women, particularly those who have been unable to conceive a longed-for child, since menopause, for them, spells the end of hope. For others, this is "no big deal", for a few it may even be a relief.

The fading of our beauty, as it is defined by our popular culture, can be a very large issue for many of us. Though we may have grumbled at times about being "just a sex object," there is an ancient, instinctual part of us which enjoys the mating dance and feels a sense of desolation when we start noticing that the men prefer dancing with younger partners. Within us all, at forty and fifty, still lives that little girl like me who wanted curly hair for the day and to dress up in her party frock and enjoy her reflection in the mirror, longing to be told she was pretty.

Aging reminds us, inevitably, that we are approaching closer to death, and for most of us, this is a scary thought. In a way, menopause, with all its little deaths—of fertility, of motherhood, of youth, etc.— is a wonderful opportunity to start rehearsing for that last great adventure, that final letting-go. But it takes courage to start thinking of it like that.

The switch from a cyclic life back to a steady state one—the dismounting from the bicycle—is one of the tasks to be accomplished. In a way, menopause is a kind of drug rehabilitation. The female body has been getting regular shots of estrogen for forty years, so it is hardly surprising that when its supply diminishes it reacts like an addict. Many menopausal symptoms are similar to opiate withdrawal.

When that withdrawal process is finally complete, our bodies feel different—lighter, the way they used to feel before we began to carry the wet heaviness of our full female anatomy and physiology. Yet they continue to carry all the memories of those wet years, distilled now into the dark sweetness of our life experience, just as raisins carry with them the essence of the grape.

Although many books have now been written about the menopausal process, one of the most important aspects which these books often neglect to mention is the need to make space for it.

Often, when something new comes into our lives, we move quickly to adjust, so that the routines to which we are accustomed now fit neatly around the new thing with minimal disruption. It is with reluctance that we give up a piece of our lives in order to accommodate the novel item, whatever it is. Even a new baby can find itself jigsawed narrowly into place between the demands of its parents' work and social schedules.

Naturally, since many of us have to earn a living, it can be hard to devote more than the minimum time to this new aspect of our inner lives. So I am not suggesting that as soon as we enter the menopause process we should drop everything and spend the next four years contemplating our navels. Few of us can afford that luxury. Just as well, really, for we need some continued interaction with the world in order to mirror the changes taking place in ourselves. What I am suggesting, however, is that this highly significant phase of our lives will be much more swiftly, successfully and thoroughly completed if we can give it some time, space and attention. Rather than brushing it aside as merely a set of physical and emotional symptoms which are nothing but a huge nuisance and an interruption of "normal" living, we are better served by embracing menopause and exploring it, for it holds many hidden treasures, not the least of which is the key to our third age and the way we are destined to live it.

For "normal" is not the life we have created, the routine that we stick to through thick and thin, the demands of the outside world upon our limited resources of time and energy. "Normal" is not the job and the commute and the in-laws, the meetings and deadlines, the annual report, the lawn to mow and the car to wash. "Normal" is the steady beating of our hearts, the rhythm of our breath, the movement of the seasons, rain on the roof, moss on stones, the behavior of birds, the cyclic progression of all living things from birth to maturity, to old age, to death, decomposition in the soil and the arising of new life. The more closely we align ourselves with that deeper sense of the "normal," the more fruitful and satisfying our lives will be. So in that sense, noticing the stirrings of the menopause process within us is a little like noticing that first faint shiver as the nights become cooler with the approach of fall and the leaves begin to lose their full summer greenness and curl up slightly at the edges. Like bears preparing for their hibernation, we need to take note and act accordingly, making space in our minds for what is happening, going with it—flowing with it.

Although the word menopause literally means the cessation of menses, I use it to signify the whole transitional period which used to be colloquially—and aptly—referred to as the "change of life." Menopause does, indeed, signify an enormous change of life. Its changes are far reaching, encompassing not only the changes in the body but a host of changes at other levels also. There are mental, emotional, psychological and spiritual components of it as well as the physical ones, and all are equally significant.

Many of the menopausal "symptoms," as I explained earlier, are similar to the familiar ones of PMS. The seesawing of emotions, the foggy brain, the lack of energy and the feelings of being back in adolescence, these will all pass, just as the hot flashes and night sweats will pass. But there are other changes which will stay with us, and deepen as we ripen further and further into our old age. The feeling of greater lightness and freedom, especially the freedom to be our true selves, will remain with us in the years that follow, as will the gradual diminishment of physical strength and stamina. Our skin will never again be plump and smooth, but will become more and more like parchment and increasingly fragile, slower to heal and marked with the signs of having lived—the clumping of pigment into age spots, which speak of all the summers we have seen, and the character lines which our living has etched upon our faces. The experiences we have collected will form the raw material of our wisdom, and the older we get, the more we shall have the courage of our own convictions.

So there are two important things to remember. One is that the temporary changes of menopause should not be confused with the permanent changes that signify the transition to becoming an elderwoman. The other is that menopause is a time when we are quite fragile. Just as a caterpillar makes a cocoon in which to undergo its metamorphosis undisturbed, so should we ensure that somewhere, somehow, we make time and space in our lives—special, private space and special, private time—to experience and explore what is going on with us, for the changes which are happening in our bodies and our psyches are every bit as far reaching as the ones which are happening to the caterpillar. And no one disturbs the caterpillar while that process is going on. The cocoon is not a luxury. It is imperative.

If we have never kept a journal, this may be the time to begin. It is a time for recording our dreams and pondering upon them; a time for expressing our feelings in words, pictures, music, shape or movement. It is a time to be a little "selfish," and put our own needs first, at least for a while. There will be as many ways of creating a cocoon as there are women, but for each of us there must be a cocoon of sorts in order for the process to complete itself and our new elderwoman's wings to form. If we neglect this all-important transition, we shall be ill-equipped to take our rightful place in society as elderwomen.

Nevertheless, life gives us ample opportunities to clear its developmental hurdles. Even when the physical symptoms of menopause have ceased, if the mental, emotional and psychological tasks have not been fully attended to, there is still time in which to complete them. If we find ourselves, at fifty-nine, still struggling with the issue of our fading petals, our drastically lowered value in the sexual marketplace, our fear of death or our regrets about our empty nests, we can still make space and deal with those issues now. We cannot move fully into our old age until they are behind us, but we have time to work at them until they are.

In fact, like the change from infant to toddler or from teenager to adult, the shift from the mother stage to the crone stage is a gradual and often blurry one. Just as spring moves into summer and summer becomes fall, there is no clear-cut moment of definition, except in terms of the rituals we ourselves create in order to honor the shift. Menopause can never be pinpointed as it happens, since we cannot (except in the event of surgery) name any bleed as our last until a year after it ceases. Only with hindsight can we say with certainty where we are.

As William Bridges pointed out many years ago in his useful little book, *Transitions*,[2] every transition has a beginning, a middle and an end. It begins with an ending. Next comes a foggy, confusing middle section, and then the end, which is a new beginning. The end of the mother phase is the beginning of menopause. It is followed by the foggy middle years, in the cocoon. Its end is the beginning of the crowning phase of our lives— our birth into elderhood.

And a birth is something to celebrate.

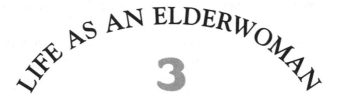

LIFE AS AN ELDERWOMAN

3

ONCE UPON A time, an old Arabian fisherman dragged a bottle out of the sea and unstoppered it, releasing a large djinn.

The djinn was murderous, rather than grateful. He said that for the first hundred years he had planned to reward whoever let him out, but in the end, sick of waiting, he became so furious that he decided to kill his rescuer instead.

The old man talked fast and managed to trick the djinn back into the bottle. End of story? No, for this is no ordinary fairy tale. This is an elder tale. In this version, the old man then sat down and started swapping stories with the captured djinn. In the end, he let him out again—and was rewarded.

Alan Chinen, a psychiatrist with a particular interest in the aging process, has made a study of fairy tales and what these have to tell us about the psychological tasks of later life.

Fairy tales—like dreams—reveal, in symbolic terms, many things which are hidden from our conscious, rational minds. Chinen's book, *In The Ever After: Fairy Tales and the Second Half of Life*, brings together a world collection of tales featuring old people as main characters. Most traditional stories, as we know, portray younger heroes and their battles, their journeys and travails and their quest for the Holy Grail in one guise or another. But these are different.

31

> *Elder tales portray a new set of virtues—wisdom, not*
> *heroism…elders affirm mediation and communication,*
> *rather than battle or conquest. Faced with the djinn, the*
> *fisherman talks and tells stories. He does not seek to*
> *destroy the monster, as the young hero typically does. The*
> *elder's role is to raise bridges, not swords.*[1]

This gentler, more conciliatory, detached and yet compassionate attitude towards what we may think of as evil is one of the chief hallmarks of the elder, in many cultures. It is a sign of wisdom. For most of us, including me, it is also one of the hardest states to attain.

This is probably why, in my search for a role model, I turned intuitively to my maternal grandmother, who seemed, to my child's eye, to personify this quality of gentleness and compassion as well as a simplicity of lifestyle with which I felt a strong affinity, even back then.

While simplicity comes easily to me, compassion is a quality I have struggled to possess, contrasting as it does with the fiery temper with which I was born and my all-too-ready tendency to judge and condemn.

Despite the fact that my personal life is relatively peaceful, I can quickly become enraged by such things as injustice, the oppression of the poor by the rich and the plunder of nature by our greedy, rapacious industrial society. I can get so infuriated about them that I block my own ability to act effectively.

During my formative years, in England, the world was at war and any moral dilemmas which previously existed resolved to black and white in the immediacy of that. Right was right and wrong was Hitler. We did our patriotic duty, knitted socks for refugees, grew vegetables, put our pocket money into National Savings Certificates to help the war effort and suffered rationing, air raids, the blackout and all other dangers and inconveniences with an expected stoicism. Then suddenly, one day, it was all over and our side had won. Thus I came into adulthood clutching the conviction that good will ultimately triumph over evil. However, my later exploration of metaphysical concepts and Eastern traditions of thought, combined with the complexities of adult life, led me gradually into a deeper, more all-inclusive, more holistic level of understanding. It was a level where good and evil are simply two sides of a coin, two parts of a whole, each playing its part in the drama and dance of life and offering us opportunities to learn and grow.

My many years of clinical practice helped, too. In our everyday lives, much of what we see of others, we see from the outside. Therapists are privileged to be invited inside. A psychotherapist needs to step outside his or her own skin, suspend personal preferences and value judgments, and enter deeply into the mind and being of the other, seeing the world through another pair of eyes. Given enough skill and empathy, it is possible to enter the world of any other human being in this intimate way, regardless of race, gender, lifestyle or circumstances, connecting at the level of shared humanity and operating from there.

I know of no other situation, except perhaps marriage, that enables—nay, demands—this primal connection and provides insight into life experiences which one could never have had for oneself. As a law-abiding, middle-class, heterosexual Englishwoman, how else could I ever, in one lifetime, have learned so much of how it felt to be a member of a racial minority, to be a man, to be poor or to be a millionaire, to be gay, to flee my country as a refugee, to live in a mansion or on the street or behind prison bars? In the act of becoming one, so to speak, with that other person, albeit only for an hour at a time, you genuinely do learn to see the world from another point of view. And the more practice you get at seeing the world from other people's points of view, the more you realize that every point of view makes perfect sense to the person holding it. Every point of view has its own internal validity, even when the world judges it bad or mad.

So being a therapist gradually made me more tolerant, more gentle, slower to judge, less certain about ultimate values. Even if I took the moral high ground because someone's actions went against established norms of right and wrong, or because I found actions like theft or murder indefensible, nevertheless my understanding of the person behind the actions taught me to condemn the actions themselves, rather than the person. In other words, it brought me to the belief that there are no intrinsically bad people, only misguided people and bad actions. It introduced me to compassion.

You may find this controversial. But I believe that it is difficult to, as Chinen suggests, "raise bridges, not swords" unless we are able somehow to cultivate the art and habit of compassion. My work as a therapist taught me compassion. There are doubtless many other ways to learn it, but learn it we must, if we are to fulfill our elderwoman role of raising bridges. This definitely does not mean being lenient with lawbreakers. It means we can be firm, uncompromising and yet kind, all at the same time. We can condemn and punish wrongdoing, while extending compassion to the wrongdoer.

Even if we learn to exercise this understanding and compassion and separate our respect for individuals from our judgment of their actions, it is still difficult not to be trapped, from time to time, into states of impotent rage against governments, corporations, or other powerful organizations and bureaucracies led by unknown and faceless "suits." This, I confess, is my personal Achilles heel. So for all of us, at various times, and in various ways, bridge-raising can be exceedingly challenging and hard.

Just as not all young people are heroes, not all old people are true elders. As Chinen says, being old is not alone enough to make us wise

> But within each person awaits the figure of the elder—a
> promise and a challenge.[2]

Each of us must meet this challenge in her own individual way and in her own unique setting. I must stress again that in order to be effective elderwomen, there is no requirement to engage in social action in the accepted sense of the word. We might never stir beyond our own living rooms or speak to more than three people in a week, and one of those might be the mail carrier. It is the way we see ourselves, the attitude to the world which we adopt, our sense of sharing in the responsibility and leadership of that world and the wisdom and compassion with which we—often without knowing it—infuse our every word and action that makes us elderwomen.

It is often the small and simple words or actions which have the greatest impact. The Grandmother's secret is that although she may appear innocent, harmless, perhaps even nondescript, she has the power to change the world, just as small green plants can push up through cement. Sometimes, she needs to do very little. In fact, her secret is more about being than about doing. Her secret is in who she is and what she stands for rather than in what she does.

My own grandmother just went about her simple daily tasks in her inimitable way, yet the lessons I learned from her were profound. And her unconditional love for me, which was deep and strong, was also of a very different nature from the love of my parents, whose responsibility it was to discipline me and bring me up in the best possible way. There was a gentle non-attachment in it. A love without strings. A love which was simply *there*.

There is a strong parallel between the loving but non-attached caring of a grandmother for her grandchildren and the loving yet non-attached caring of the elderwoman for the wellbeing of her society and the overall welfare of the Earth. An elderwoman who does have grandchildren will be expressing this caring at both personal and planetary levels at the same time.

To whatever extent a woman has family around her who look to her as their senior member, she will be performing a moral leadership role, either overtly, like a matriarch, or subtly, the way my own grandmother did. And Grandma's way was so subtle that I cannot even describe how she did it. She never lectured or preached. Most of her moralizing came in the form of her pithy little sayings—which usually hit the spot. But she was a moral leader, nonetheless.

Leadership, in our modern consumer culture, has been hijacked by corporate power and, instead of resting in the hands of the elders, as it did for millennia, it is now given into the hands of the twenty- thirty- and forty-somethings, most of whom grew up with the information technology which has assisted that corporate domination. But there is another force which is gathering momentum, the voice of the "cultural creatives," the fifty million people in America who sociologist Paul H. Ray and psychologist Sherry Ruth Anderson refer to—based on their thirteen years of research—as the leading-edge creators of a new culture. They are the ones whose core values are unrelated to the dominant paradigm of expansion and consumption, and who care more about the quality of being than the rat race of getting and having.

Ray and Anderson describe this group as caring deeply about ecology and saving the planet, about relationships, peace, social justice, and about self-actualization, spirituality and self-expression. They are people who are both inner directed and socially concerned. Many are activists for one cause or another. But most are unaware of just how large a group they really are.

*Once they realize their numbers, their impact on American
life promises to be enormous, shaping a new agenda for the
twenty-first century.*[3]

It is estimated by these researchers that as well as the fifty million
cultural creatives in the U.S.A., there are a further eighty to ninety million
in Europe. A large proportion are women. Many are, or will become,
elderwomen. In fact, you could say that the elderwoman is either a cultural
creative who has reached the third age of her life or a woman who has
become a cultural creative as she ages.

So it is in recognition of the latent power in coming generations of
grandmothers that this book is written. In the chapters that follow, I want
to take us on a wide-ranging journey through many areas of the
elderwoman's life.

Each of our lives will be different in form and content, since we are all
individuals. So I make no attempt to prescribe the exact details of how we
should live. My intent is to articulate a vision of the elderwoman and the
sorts of things which may be important to her. It is more of an artist's
impression than a detailed photograph.

As a way of ensuring some sort of wholeness for this work, I have
chosen the ancient concept of elements as a way of structuring its contents
and of looking at some facets of the elderwoman's relationship with the
world. So let me briefly remind you of that concept.

If you trace back the history of Western science to it roots in ancient
Greece, you find that an early attempt to explain how this world was put
together was a dividing of all matter into four elements: earth, air, fire and
water.

In the East, the system was more complex. The original,
undifferentiated whole from which all existence was born was called the
Tao. The Tao was so complete and undifferentiated that it could not be
visualized or conceptualized except in the most abstract way. By definition,
it was beyond the grasp of the finite human mind. As the ancient sage Lao
Tzu explained, the Tao which could be named was not the Tao. In other
words, if you think you have understood it, that isn't it!

This primal wholeness became two forces, the force of yin and the
force of yang, and all of matter, all of existence, could be explained in terms
of the interplay of these two. When they combined in certain ways, other

elements came into existence, the primary ones—earth, air, fire, water—
and secondary ones such as metal and wood. Played upon by the eternal
flow of *chi* (spirit), these elements combined in countless millions of subtly
different ways to create "The Ten Thousand Things," (everything in
existence).

This book draws on both Eastern and Western concepts. Chapters 4
through 23 are in sections corresponding to the four elements, as follows:

- **Earth is our place of belonging.** First, we explore the earth forces by
  looking at such issues as the significance of the soil itself as a
  foundation for life, our relationship to our home planet and its
  creatures, and the importance of grounding in our emotional and
  spiritual lives.

- **Air is the element of lightness and freedom.** So in this section, we
  consider such matters as the lightening of our materiality as we age
  and the lightness of our footprints on the Earth.

- **Fire is the element of passion,** and that which gives heart and
  meaning to our lives. It is red, the color of blood. So in this section we
  talk about love, kinship, relationship and the various forms of passion,
  personal and political.

- **Water is the element of fluidity,** the principle of constant, universal
  change and flow. Here, we look at the flow of our own lives, and their
  totality, from infancy to old age, as though each life is a river, heading
  towards the ocean.

Yin and yang are explored in Chapters 24 through 28, as we turn to the
question of balance in all aspects of our lives.

Another aspect of balance, which permeates the whole book, is the
need to be aware of both our inner and outer lives, balancing outward
action with inner contemplation.

One of the key concepts in this book is the attainment of simplicity.
And I have attempted to create balance here also: prescriptions for
simplifying consumption patterns, habits, food, clothes, vacations—you
name it—are not enough on their own. But neither is it sufficient to be
inspired by ideas, without reference to how these might work in practice.
Changes are most successful if they happen at both inner and outer levels
at the same time.

When my desk is cluttered, my mind is cluttered. And a cluttered, overfull, bursting-at-the-seams mind tends to create a collection of stuff around us. When our insides (minds) are crowded, our outsides (desks, lives, diaries) are crowded, and vice versa. When we live in a busy, busy world, we become busier and busier. The outside affects the inside, and pretty soon you are in a vicious circle. Therefore, any attempt to simplify must address both inside and outside simultaneously. So balancing inside and outside is a theme which you will find running through the book.

Let's start on our journey, now, through the elements. And as we go, we shall seek out the key principles on which the elderwoman's life is based.

Simplicity is one of my favorites, and you will find that recurring in various parts of the book. So is the art of seeing beneath the surface, both into our deeper selves and into the mind and motivations of another. I call this the principle of deep vision. This leads to a third, which is compassion. Together with the fourth principle—non-attachment—we achieve the ability to raise bridges, in just the way that Chinen and the elder tales are stressing. For as he says:

> The most challenging task of later life can be said to be
> uniting inner exploration and social benefit.[4]

Here, then, are the first four principles of the elderwoman's life:

• simplicity • deep vision • compassion • non-attachment •

Let's proceed, and see what others we can find.

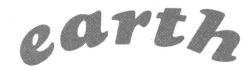

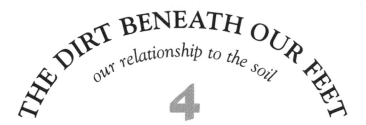

THE DIRT BENEATH OUR FEET

our relationship to the soil

4

LIKE MANY older women, then and now, my grandmother was a keen gardener. When I was five, she donated a little patch of her garden to me, and gave me sunflower seeds to plant. For ages, nothing happened. Then, tiny shoots appeared. I watched in amazement as the plants grew and grew until they were more than twice as tall as me, their huge yellow heads nodding over, way above my head. It seemed like a miracle. Well, it was, really.

Back then, I assumed that soil was just inert stuff that held the roots and supported the plant stems. No one told me otherwise. It was many years before I really understood what an amazing and important substance soil is, and how unappreciated and badly treated it is by some sections of humanity. Only quite recently did I realize how much it needs our care and understanding. It dawned on me that the elderwoman is one of the soil's chief guardians. A good relationship with it can, in turn, enrich her life, which is why I want to begin this contemplation of the earth element by thinking about it very literally.

Dirt, soil, earth. The topsoil, the subsoil, the rock underneath. All our lives, we rest upon it. Depend upon it, literally, in all senses of the word. Yet If you think about it, we modern folk spend very little time with our feet actually touching the earth itself. Some of us might go a whole day without glimpsing bare soil. We can even forget that it exists. Much of the time, especially if we live in the city, between that soil and our feet lies the dead weight of concrete, sitting dully and heavily over soil which may never see the sun again. That always makes me feel sad. Although I know it is a silly fantasy, since builders always remove the topsoil before they build, I still have this image of some poor mole or earthworm struggling to the surface only to discover he or she has come up right under the middle of Safeway or the Interstate or Gate Fifteen of the airport. It is a dilemma, for I need stores and roads and airports, too, just like everybody else does. I also need the soil, for my life utterly depends upon it. Without soil, there would be no food, and without food we would all die. So it seems important to me to think about this dirt, this thing that one's life depends on.

Firstly, I believe we need to think about it in order to ensure that it is being properly taken care of and that there is enough of it that is *not* covered over. Lots of areas where the trees can grow and the moles and earthworms can still poke through the surface. And lots of it that never will be covered over—ever. Because land developers and builders—and governments—often don't notice when they are overdoing things and putting profit ahead of health and sanity. Sometimes it needs older people to point this out; people who have been around a long time and who can see the long-term effects of things are the ones who need to speak out. Just as longitudinal studies in science are a particularly useful and valid way of gaining information, the voices and opinions of older people in a society have a value all their own. It is we who remember the green field which predated a certain parking lot, cattle grazing in what is now the shopping mall, the chopped-down trees. It is we who need to cry out "STOP!" and make our voices heard, for we are the only ones who truly understand what is being lost.

Secondly, I think we need to look at our relationship with the soil from the point of view of having been created out of it, and being headed towards intimate reunion with it after our death. Realizing the importance of that relationship, in our third age we might want to put more emphasis on celebrating that deep connection. We might want to find opportunities in our lives to walk barefoot, to dig in the garden, plant things in the soil, smell it, get it on our hands. There is literally an earthy satisfaction for many of us in those things, a satisfaction which we may have forgotten in our busy lives up among the concrete buildings, and which will come flooding back when we walk barefoot along the beach or spend an afternoon on our knees in the garden, weeding and planting and mulching.

And as we age, and begin to think more often about our own death, there can be a certain special comfort in remembering our intimate relationship with the soil.

Thirdly, it seems important to consider the symbolic aspect of it. In other words, the necessity to stay grounded. Physically, we do this by remaining aware of our bodies and not ignoring or overriding their messages of weariness or pain. This becomes increasingly important as we age, for our powers of recuperation are slower and less efficient. Emotionally, we do it by keeping a firm hold on reality and commonsense and by tempering drama with humor. And spiritually, we do it by honoring our legacy as wisdomkeepers, members of an ancient lineage of women with a special relationship to nature.

So, if the bodies we live in are actually constructed out of the earth, and earth is the substance on which our life and existence depends, surely it must be a highly important substance? Something to give some thought to. What actually *is* it? Why does it do often get treated as dispensable, as insignificant—or even as horrible? ("Dirt"—"dirty"—"disgusting.")

I remember thinking about that one day, nearly six years ago, after I had been standing in an airport departure lounge, watching a grandson—then not quite a year old—toddling around on the floor, trying out this new mode of locomotion so lately learned.

I recall the way his curved, pink baby feet struggled to splay flat and hold his body vertical. He stepped, he wobbled, he collapsed. Tried again, collapsed, gave up, returned to crawling mode.

This he could do, of course, with the speed of several months intensive practice. So off he went, skimming across the vast acres of polished airport vinyl, dodging the travelers and their suitcases. He reached a large trash can of cylindrical metal, twice his height. Up went the hands, fingers seeking, exploring. On to his feet again then, stretching up, those little fingers curling over the top of the trash can, gripping, pulling, until down it came, in a shower of cigarette ash, apple cores, Styrofoam cups and candy wrappers. He settled down contentedly, amid his booty, keen to examine every new object, perhaps to taste some.

By the time I retrieved him, his pink hands and feet and knees were a grimy gray and I tucked him on to my hip and raced for the washroom as though the seeds of a dozen weird and possibly fatal diseases were waiting only for him to put a finger in his mouth.

As I held him firmly with one arm around his waist and used my free hand to wash those baby fingers, my mind went back one week. We had been in the country, staying in a small cabin that my friend Daphne owns.

There he was, in my memory's eye, crawling to the edge of the cabin doorway and easing himself gently over the step. There he was, crawling across the uneven brick paving, pausing to examine and to taste the weeds that grew between the cracks, to pick up a small stone, to dabble in the untidy place where paving and grass met, their boundary blurred by the sprawl of alyssum and nasturtiums.

Off he scuttled, emboldened by a quick look behind him to check that his mother and I were still waiting and caring; off to the mysteries of rainwater tank and bucket, of rock and log, of soft leaves and prickly leaves, darting skinks and slow-moving beetles, and above all, of earth. Dark brown earth.

I remember him coming back, his knees now green from grass, fragments of soil and sand in the soft crevices of his plump little hands, and I remember how I scooped him up and fed him some mashed carrots on a spoon and then, after a while, returned him to his mother's breast for refreshment and sleep, and none of us even thought of washing him. So what was the difference? He was dirty, but this time it didn't matter. Why not? What, then, *is* dirt? Words like "dirty" and "soiled" seem to denote some unhealthy, unpleasant state of being, a contamination.

It was only after the airport incident that the truth came to me. The truth that there must once have been a time when the only way you got dirty was in the dirt. The only way you got soiled was in the soil. There was no other class of dirt except that which lay on the forest floor of our ancestors, or within the caves they used for shelter.

The soil, then as now, was made up of three basic types of ingredients: minerals (the fragmentary particles of all kinds of rocks), humus and living organisms. The humus was composed of a vast conglomeration of once-living matter, the waste products of creatures, the broken down remnants of plant parts, all combined into a rich, nurturing compound, essential to continuing life. It was from this compound that seedlings drew their nourishment and built themselves into grass, flowers, trees—green and growing things which, in their turn, nourished and built the animals. Organisms living within this soil mixture—molds, bacteria, worms and other creatures—made up the huge army of workers that converted the raw materials, like dead plant and animal matter, human and animal wastes, etc., into usable form. A huge army which, by the way, is still largely unstudied. Daphne, who studied microbiology at college, informed me recently that only a mere 5 percent of soil organisms have ever been described and classified even though there are thousands of different kinds in every teaspoonful of soil. I thought this was pretty amazing. I always assumed that scientists knew everything there was to know about soil, but apparently their knowledge is extremely limited.

Once all these decaying and putrefying materials are fully decomposed and turned into humus, they are sweet smelling, clean, beautiful and wholesome again. They eventually become the crumbly chocolate-colored compost into which we love to plant our daffodil bulbs.

But between the decaying, rotting matter and the sweet smelling compost there is a time gap—and, for most of us, an awareness gap. The process of transformation is slow and mysterious and takes place mostly in the dark. So we see the two ends of the cycle but not the middle. Unless, like Daphne, we recycle everything ourselves. Then we see the whole cycle. But most of us do not live like Daphne. We throw our garbage in the bin and we buy the compost at the garden store and we rarely if ever think about what lies between these two events.

When I rushed my grandson to the airport washroom, the dirt on his little pink hands seemed menacing somehow, ugly, out of place, obscene. It seemed to contain the dirt of a thousand feet that had walked who knows where, over who knows what. The noxious mixture from the trash can was the raw detritus of a culture that no longer recognizes the existence of its own waste products, let alone honors and recycles them. And many are not recyclable anyway. Therefore, this unknown mixture on his innocent hands repulsed and terrified me at some unconscious level where I intuitively felt—rather than thought about—the difference.

Around that cabin, on the other hand, things lived and things died, and everything, even peoples' own waste products, ended up eventually as sweet smelling compost in the garden or the orchard. (Daphne explained that the residue from the composting toilets only goes into the orchard, and not on the vegetable patch, and I must admit I found that reassuring.) The process may be mysterious and wonderful, but the processed components are known. We always knew what went in, and always knew what came out. Daily, we remembered to bless the seen and unseen army of converters, the earthworms and their zillions of smaller companions that thrive beneath the surface of our soil. The child, crawling there, was crawling in the known world. Lightly guarded by those who know which berries and which spiders to watch out for, he was safe in his adventuresome exploration of the earth. So I think that quality of familiarity with the earth, with the movement of things in and out of it, is something we have largely lost. Our loss of that familiarity and knowing, and the pollution of the soil by umpteen industrial and commercial processes that we know so little of, has separated us from that which is really the matrix of our existence. It has made us strangers to the soil and made of dirt a foreign and potentially lethal substance. In a way, we have become strangers to ourselves—to our own bodies and to their matrix.

The soil, and the rock below it, is the body of the Earth. The body with which we were born and in which we age is our borrowed piece of soil. We leave it behind us when we die, returning it to whence it came. So to me it makes sense that while it is in our care, we take good care of it. Like a library book, we should not trash it. Similarly, it behooves us to take good care of the Earth's body too, since everything else which lives depends on that. To me, there is a deep connection between the way we take care of our bodies and the way we take care of the soil and of the world. Start thinking about one, follow it far enough and it inevitably leads you to thoughts of the other two. Want to be more healthy? Improve your diet. Which means eat better quality, cleaner food—organic food. Which means healthier soil. Which means a healthier planet.

Most books on advice about aging remind you to take good care of your health. I have never seen one yet which mentioned soil except maybe to suggest that gardening is a nice hobby for the retirement years. But as I have tried to show in this chapter, soil is part of the elderwoman's story. Our bodies are the soil, they are the Earth. As the Irish philosopher John O'Donohue so lyrically expresses it, we are beings made of clay.

> *We so easily forget that our clay has a memory that preceded our minds, a life of its own before it took its present form. Regardless of how modern we seem, we still remain ancient, sisters and brothers of the one clay… The human body is at home on the earth.*[1]

As I mentioned before, there is a symbolic level to all this too. As elderwomen, we contain within our collective unconscious many ancient mysteries of the soil. Even though we may be only dimly aware of it, we hold a legacy of lore and folk wisdom, a knowledge of herbs and healing, an understanding of natural processes which has been handed down from woman to woman over millennia. Much of it has gone out of sight, deep underground, some through persecution, some through the bulldozer of scientific rationalism. But as part of society's "bedrock," every elderwoman is a guardian of that ancient legacy. And in many forms and many places she is gradually bringing it out again into the light and holding it up to be honored once again. So whether or not each of us, personally, has any factual knowledge about folk medicine or herbs or healing, we all share in the symbolic guardianship of this legacy. It is the legacy of elderwomen, worldwide. There is nothing in particular that we need to do about this. We simply need to acknowledge it to ourselves and recognize it in each other when we glimpse it.

It is no accident that so many of us, in our elder years, derive such pleasure from growing things, whether in a large garden or a few pots on the windowsill. Since we are, more than any other group in this society, the official guardians of the sacred aspects of soil, gardening is one of the ways we worship.

So when the grandchildren plant sunflowers in my garden, one spring soon, I shall have a lot to tell them. About the importance of soil, and the creatures who live in it. About the importance of nurturing and protecting it, for all our human sakes and for the sakes of all those non-human life forms with whom we share the planet. About its sacred nature.

I shall explain about humus. And about the huge, unthanked workforce of indefatigable beings who create the basis for new life out of the raw materials of death. A healthy patch of soil, I shall point out to the children, is a huge, complex ecosystem in itself. An underground community. A vast co-operative project undertaken by billions and billions of tiny interdependent creatures, most of whom we neither see nor know the names of. All of them matter.

I hope the children listen. And when one day, quite a few years from now, that grandson who pulled over the trashcan takes his own suitcase and walks through the airport towards a wider world, I hope he remembers the soil beneath the concrete and the creatures of the earth. I hope they are still there for him, in even greater numbers, as people gradually begin to remember the importance of soil, of dirt, of earth. And I hope there are many days in his man's life when that soil is sweet upon his hands and rich beneath his fingernails.

From this contemplation of the soil in both its physical and symbolic aspects, we can gather up another elderwoman principle. Combining a personal quality of groundedness with the elderwoman's inherited function as guardian of the bedrock of her culture, adding her respect for the soil and its creatures, and her identification with the planet itself (which I shall speak more about in the next chapter), we find ourselves with a fifth principle which I shall call Earth-centeredness.

• simplicity • deep vision • compassion • non-attachment • Earth-centeredness •

So, with that now added to our list, let's turn to the whole question of where we live and what our relationship might be to that dwelling place.

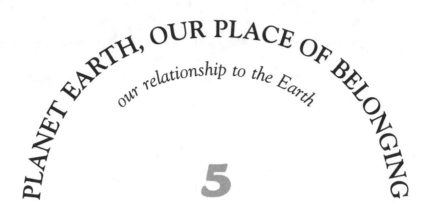

PLANET EARTH, OUR PLACE OF BELONGING

our relationship to the Earth

5

WHAT DOES the word "home" mean to you?

Maybe you would like to put the book down and spend a few moments pondering that question, for it could be a rather important one.

For many of us, this issue becomes especially significant during the later years of our lives, particularly if we have roamed the world, moved house many times and are no longer quite sure where our true home might be. The majority of us, after all, are likely find ourselves grounded for our very final years. So this may be our last chance to get it right and live in the place that feels best to us. Or we may be forced to accept that we never shall. In which case, we have to grieve the loss of a long-held dream and get on with building, instead, a relationship to the place in which we find ourselves.

Some people seek out warmer climates in which to rest elderly bones. Others remain attached to much loved houses and hope to stay in them to the end, among familiar things and routines, friends and neighbors. Some move closer to sons and daughters, or to particular services—a church, a hospital—anticipating lessened mobility and perhaps a need for care. Others book themselves into communities specifically tailored to the needs of the old. To some, location is unimportant. This could be because they are equally happy anywhere, or because—anticipating an after-life—they see a temporal home as a temporary place. It might be because the people they are with are more important to them than the place itself. Or maybe they have resigned themselves to a fate in which they have no further say.

An elderwoman may fall into any of these categories—or none. But one thing which marks her out from others is her deeper sense of the relationship between person and planet; her sense of what home really means, both to her personally and to our species as a whole.

Much as I love the term Mother Earth, in a way I see that metaphor of motherhood as slightly misleading. Sure, to the extent that a child is formed out of the mother's body, each of us is made from the substance of the Earth. However, a child is always destined to grow up and move away from its mother. Whereas we, as parts of Earth herself, cannot ever move away from her, which is where the mother-child metaphor falls down.

The way I prefer to think of it is that we are more like cells of the Earth's body—mobile ones, like individual, separate blood corpuscles, forever moving around within her, dying off and being re-absorbed.

So if we are an integral part of the Earth, then why and how have we come to the point where our species is trashing it? Ecological philosopher Paul Shepard maintained that the problem began many thousands of years ago, with the start of agriculture.[1] He believed that our hunter-gatherer forebears, who moved around and gained their sustenance from the environment as a whole, would have had no feeling of separateness from it. They were so enveloped in—and nourished by—the environment that they had no sense of it as "not-self," just as a fish is so utterly enveloped in water that it would have no concept of "water" until someone tried to pull it out of the stream.

According to Shepard, once people began to save seeds, settle in villages and domesticate animals, they began to be more affected by the problem of good years and bad years. Nature came to be seen as a mother. Sometimes she was benevolent and harvests were good, but sometimes she appeared punishing and withholding. Gradually, over the centuries which followed, this led to a battle mentality and to a situation where man [sic] became constantly at war with nature, struggling endlessly to dominate and vanquish her. In our own times, this insane, slow matricide continues unabated, despite the obvious truth that if it succeeds, all life on Earth is doomed.

All of us in the Western world have been brought up in a culture permeated with this alienated attitude. We have soaked in its ideas without realizing it. It is impossible not to. True Earth wisdom, based on a full identification with the Earth is something we in our Western techno-culture have to regain, slowly and painfully. To regain it, most of us have to call into question virtually everything we have been taught and apprentice ourselves instead to a new set of teachers—to the trees and the stars and the cycle of seasons, to the animals without and the animal within. We have to listen to our own inner knowing and also to admit the depth of our own ignorance.

Inasmuch as the elderwoman is a key representative of Earth wisdom, she faces the task of re-interpreting all her acquired ideas, her lifestyle and her words and actions in the light of this wisdom, which takes some doing. The good news, though, is that this wisdom was never really lost. It was only buried. So if we seek it, we shall find it. And we shall find it right here. Since we all carry the genes of our hunter-gatherer ancestors, we also carry their intuitive wisdom about the true nature of our relationship with our world. As Shepard says,

> *Hidden from history, this secret person is undamaged in each of us and may be called forth by the most ordinary acts of life.*[2]

To rediscover the "secret person" who is in tune with the Earth, it is only necessary to listen and look deeply, around us and within us. At this stage of our lives, we can no longer claim that we do not have time for that. It can be—and should be—a high priority now. Old age is designed to accommodate such things. And for many of us, that deep listening is often aided by certain experiences—moments of sudden insight, particularly in natural settings, which bring with them a new and profound understanding.

Some places seem especially conducive to this type of occurrence. Just as the true elderwoman is a human conduit for wisdom, certain spots on the Earth's surface are conduits also. Some natural power spots—like the famous vortices of Sedona, Arizona—are like acupuncture points on the surface of the Earth, places of fine, clear and extraordinary energy where the air itself almost crackles. Others, like Stonehenge or Chartres Cathedral, are places where centuries of reverence have created a special patina. The air in those places does not so much crackle as sing. In those places, insights come to us effortlessly, as though breathed in with that very air.

Each of us, too, has her own personal sacred place or places, places to which we go for inspiration, nourishment, comfort or communion. These are the places which our souls recognize as home. And it is in these places the insights are often more likely to arise, since there our minds are more likely to be open and receptive than they are anywhere else.

The places which are personally significant to us—our own sacred sites—are not necessarily located in remote rural areas, though for many they are. I know someone whose moment of greatest inspiration happened in a suburban street, as she looked at a flower in someone's garden. For some people, no sound but birdsong or the trickling of a stream over stones can create a sacred space, and my friend Parvati is convinced that anything more must surely "block the energy" as she puts it, but I know full well that there are people whose souls can be stirred, just as easily as hers, against the roar and bustle of Piccadilly or Times Square. Conversely, there are wonderful natural places—Niagara Falls being a good example—where for me it is a struggle to make contact with the sacred element of place because of the thick layer of crass commercialism which surrounds them. (In visiting such places, it is worth making the extra effort to get up early and try to get there before the crowds arrive, as my family and I did on the magical morning at Delphi which I tell about in Chapter 9).

I recall a long trek I once made up a hot and dusty canyon to see an ancient and remote cliff dwelling in Arizona, and how wonderful it was, as our small group stood there taking in the awesome experience of that site, to have our guide request silence. I felt like hugging him. For idle chatter in such a special place can pain the ear in the same way that graffiti on a beautiful building can pain the eye.

Wonderful as it is to visit these places of special significance, the most important way in which we connect with our Earth is by deepening our relationship with the ordinary, everyday places in which we live, and in particular, tuning in to whatever parts of them still move according to the seasonal cycles of nature, even if that is only a patch of grass which turns brown in winter and green again in summer, pigeons nesting on a ledge, or a harvest moon rising over downtown skyscrapers.

For me, although I love the countryside best, there are certain cities and towns which feel special to me. If a city, no matter how large, has places in it that are human-sized and human-shaped, and is imprinted with centuries of ordinary, low-tech human living and interaction, it can feel benign and pleasant. Alleyways, cobblestones, window boxes full of geraniums, pedestrian-only precincts, sidewalk cafes, old inns—these for me are features of delight. In the same way, I delight in the ancient flagstones of my own cottage floor, worn by three centuries of feet, and in the fact that I can place my hand upon my living room ceiling without standing on tiptoes. I would not swap my wood stove for central heating, my old scarred floorboards for luxury carpet or my secondhand furniture for the latest fashion. But these are personal preferences. For some people, life in a small cottage with one bathroom would induce more claustrophobia than delight. An eagle could not live comfortably in a rabbit hole and a prairie dog alone on a rocky ledge would pine to death. There are many definitions of specialness, of sacredness, and of what it is that really feels like home.

One of my favorite anecdotes is the one told by a returning American astronaut who described his excitement, shortly after take-off, at being able to see his entire home state at a glance. A while later, he realized, with fascination, that he could now see the entire American continent. "There's my home," he thought in wonderment. But as the spacecraft moved farther and farther away from the Earth's surface, finally that moment came when he could see the entire planet framed in the porthole, like some glorious blue and gold jewel suspended in the velvet darkness of space. "There's my home," he whispered, awestruck. In that moment, he said later, his whole life changed.

It is unlikely that many of us will travel far enough to see what that man saw. But we can, like most other creatures, locate within ourselves a feeling of identification with home. Many creatures never travel more than a few miles—or even mere inches—from where they were born. Of those who do travel, most follow the same routes and return again and again to that particular spot on the Earth's surface which they call home. A returning salmon, after an ocean journey of thousands of kilometers, finds once again the mouth of the river, and swims up it until she finds that very patch of river pebbles over which her own life began. How she does this, no one knows. It is one of the great unsolved mysteries, along with the ability of swallows to return to the same telegraph wires, homing pigeons to fly unerringly to their lofts, or monarch butterflies to cross huge continents and land in the exact same tree, year after year.

Do we, too, have a similar instinct, perhaps largely lost or submerged, to create a connection like that with one piece of the Earth's surface and return to it whenever we have wandered? I believe some of us do, and it seems likely that some do not. I have met many people who were never happy in their home town, or native land, and eventually found a completely different place which felt far more like home to them. I have met people who feel equally at home anywhere. Like Kipling's Cat That Walked by Himself, all places are alike to them. They are planetary citizens.

At one time I believed that an identification with the whole planet as a personal home was in some way spiritually superior to a more localized sense of home. I imagined that someone who had seen the Earth from space would henceforth be content to live anywhere. That belief made my own private obsession with finding just the right spot for myself—a quest which took me more than half a century—seem somehow ignoble and petty. What I did not understand, back then, was that an identification of myself as an integral part of the planet was still perfectly compatible with a desire to find my special place.

It took me years to grasp it, but for me the message of the astronaut's story was not only that he recognized Earth as his home, but that when he saw each level of home he discovered that they nested inside each other, like Matryoshka dolls.

Children instinctively understand this nested reality. Is there any one of us who has not, at some point in our childhood, written our name and address then, after the zip code and our home country, added "The World... The Solar System... The Milky Way... The Universe?"

For some people, this sense of complete belonging to the Earth is incompatible with religious belief. Our soul's home, they believe, is not here but elsewhere. And it is true that even within those who, like me, have sought and found our special place, and experience contentment there, a deep and unexplained longing for homecoming can still occasionally prevail. It is a kind of soul hunger, a "homesickness for the divine," which cannot be satisfied by geographical relocation.

This used to puzzle me until I remembered that as a child I was taught that heaven was elsewhere. It suddenly dawned on me that if I am part of the Earth then my soul, too, is part of a greater soul. Heaven, surely, is not another place, but simply another dimension of this one. And the divine homesickness which comes over us at times—perhaps more so as we age— may simply be a longing to move into that other dimension where there is no longer anything about us that feels separate.

A while ago, with that feeling in mind, I wrote a sonnet about the stream which runs through the bottom of the valley near my house. In the southwest of England, where I live, these tiny valleys are called combes, and each one runs through fields and woods and finally empties out into the ocean just as, at death, we empty out again into that primal oneness with all things. Here is what I wrote:

FINAL MOMENTS

In blind return to the Atlantic womb,
This eager stream has furrowed to the shore,
Through green, sheep-sprinkled, Devon hills, a combe
Lush lined with oak and beech and sycamore.

Deep in this fold, her journey's legacy
Of silt to ferns bequeathed, her life's tales told,
She flows with softness, equanimity.
Her waters light; no burden left to hold.

Suddenly, now! She rounds the combe's last bend
A dozen yards from where the breakers crash.
The last tree passed. Salt stings the air. The end.
Time now to make that final, trembling dash

Through hard, gray rock, where gulls scream at the sun,
Die to herself, and open to the One.

So what really *is* "home" then?

Is it a particular house? A room, a special chair, a garden? Is it a neighborhood, a town? A certain fork in childhood's favorite tree?

Is it the body in which our soul is temporarily resident? Is it people? A family? The arms of a lover?

Is it a state or a country? Is it Planet Earth? Is it the infinite Universe? Is it that unknown, all-encompassing something that some call God?

The answer is easy. It is all of the above. It simply depends where your spacecraft happens to be, any time you look out of the porthole.

As elderwomen, there is an inclusiveness, now, in the way we see everything. We are beginning to have a holistic view. This is yet another aspect of that principle I call deep vision. Not only do we understand that the Universe is composed of systems within systems, but we are learning to shift focus from one system to another as required without losing our sense of the whole picture. This is deep vision at its most developed. The elderwoman can move up and down the scale as necessary. She can switch in a second from the contemplation of far galaxies to playing peek-a-boo with her youngest grandchild. Her deep vision is both telescope and microscope, encompassing both the vast and the miniscule. It can spread sideways in all directions to rest on the others who share the planet with her. And it is to this we shall turn next, as we consider our relationships with the landscape, then with other human beings, with other non-human creatures and with non-living objects.

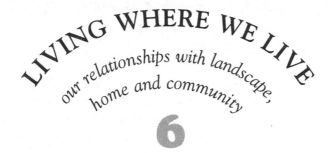

LIVING WHERE WE LIVE
our relationships with landscape, home and community

6

IF I GO TO THE topmost window in my house or the highest point of my garden, I can almost see the ocean. Not quite, but I know it is there, and if I walk for forty-five minutes I can stand at the top of the cliffs, watching the waves break on the rocks below. I get an immense feeling of pleasure and satisfaction from this simple fact.

When I was a child, I lived a similar distance from the ocean and on a clear day I could see it just. And in my first solo apartment, at twenty-three, there was one window from which, if I stood on a chair, I could see the ocean—a different ocean that time.

It seems like coincidence. Yet probably it is not. For all of us, there are certain configurations of landscape which spell "home," for many, many reasons, but most of those have their origins on our childhood experience. I recently met a woman whose parents had taken her, as a baby, to live in the Australian outback. When they returned, years later, to the small harborside town where she was born, she recoiled in horror at the sight of the tiny houses, crowding closely around the shoreline—a sight which others find charming and picturesque. How could anyone, she wondered, live without the wide, empty spaces, the desert and the endless sky? She pined for Australia until she was old enough to return there on her own, for only there could she feel at home.

Our feelings are connected with place, with landscape and with the objects around us. As Clare Cooper Marcus explains it, since feelings occur in space, naturally they tend to be associated with the place in which they occurred. Thus, emotion and place

> *are inexplicably connected, not in a causal*
> *relationship, but in a transactional exchange, unique to*
> *each person.*[1]

Researching for her book, *House as a Mirror of Self: exploring the deeper meaning of home*, rather than simply interviewing people in the normal way, Marcus invited each interview subject to draw a picture of his or her house and then to place the drawing in a chair, as though it were another person, and dialog with it. The results were fascinating. They revealed the amazing depth to which our chosen residences reflect our inner selves and the extent to which we will go to create a dwelling-place exactly suited to our needs. This often involves an unconscious replication of those things which gave us the greatest pleasure or comfort in our childhood. The author herself, who, like me, is English by birth, found herself recreating the English garden of her childhood in her backyard in Berkeley, California, just as I once tried to create one in the middle of the Australian bush without realizing—until later, when severe drought had killed off all my roses—what I was actually doing.

The architect, Christopher Alexander, who has tried to take the designing of shelter out of the iron grip of professional architects and return it to ordinary people, speaks of how important it is for young couples to be able to co-create a house along with a relationship. Rather than buying a new house, they should find a place that they can change gradually over the years, thereby "tuning it to their lives." He, too, is talking about this notion of a transactional relationship between feeling and place and pointing out that it is linked, also, to our developmental stages.[2]

What are the implications of all this for the elderwoman? Our third age is a time for paring down to the very essentials of who we are, for throwing out excess baggage and expressing, in every aspect of our lives, the core qualities of our own individual selves. If we have partners, the chances are that we shall have a good sense now of how our needs and preferences can mesh and be accommodated within the same shared space. For those of us who have been nomadic, it is often a time when we slow down and come to rest. And it is the beginning of a time when, as in childhood, our dependence upon others may once again become paramount. So our choice of landscape, home and community is a crucial one.

This may be the last chance we have to ensure, if we can, that the landscape in which we now find ourselves is one which resonates deeply in our souls. And if it is not, then we need to mourn that loss and to do what we can to bring in that missing element in some symbolic form. (This reminds me of something long forgotten. During one particular four year stretch of my life when I lived miles from the water, there was a huge painting of ocean waves on my living room wall!) The more successfully we do that, the better we shall be at adapting to the reality of our less-than-ideal surroundings and making a real relationship with the place we are in.

It is important to ensure that if any elderly relatives—or we ourselves—ever face the need to move into residential care, such as a nursing home, the space be personalized to the greatest extent possible with the beloved objects and symbolic statements of that person's life. Home does not have to be big. It can be as small as a cubicle. But it has to be unique and has to be made to feel as close to perfect for its individual occupant as it possibly can, reflecting not only that person's life but also his or her favorite landscapes.

Along with home and landscape, we need to consider community and neighborhood. Our relationship to these, too, often has its origins in our childhood experience.

Still vivid in my memory is a picture of the street where I lived out my first nine years. Not only the street itself, but the folks who shared it. Like Mrs. G next door, with her flowery apron and her rather stern expression and the pots of runny marmalade she liked to make. Most of all, of course, I remember which houses had kids in them. Jean, at the bottom of the hill, Jimmy two doors down, Bobby across the other side, Winnie at the top.

Our neighbors, along with our families and our friends, are the people who help to shape us. They are the ones with whom we share the everyday adventures. But their importance to us fluctuates, according to the stages of our lives. When I think back to my shifting, roaming twenties, to the years of commuting from apartment to office, I have few, if any, memories of local community from that era. Not until my own children were born and my daily world shrank once more to the immediate locality, did neighborhood once more become important. I remember how eagerly, then, I sought out the other young mothers. We passed each other, wheeling our babies, holding our erratically wandering toddlers by the hand. Eyes met. We smiled, exchanged the first shy greetings. Soon we were visiting each other's houses for cups of coffee, our children scrambling together on the rug. Life had come full circle. Ask my daughters for their memories and they will tell you of the kids in *their* street alongside whom they graduated from scrambling on the rug to playing in the park, walking to school, going off to college. Helena next door, Wayne, Lynne and Philip three doors to the left, Tony across the way…

And now that I am old, neighborhood is even more important. One day, it may be essential. Many of us will end our days alone, perhaps confined to the house or to the chair. When that time comes, we can only survive if there are people around to help us. Without organic community, the kind which we have drawn around us and which can support us to the end, we shall have to move into a community of a different, less personal kind, i.e. an institution.

So community, neighborhood, friends and neighbors—all these seem increasingly precious to me now. When I walk down the main street of my village and people greet me by name, it brings a cozy glow to my heart. A sense of belonging, and a sense of gratitude that this, my community, holds me within its circle and gives me plenty of opportunities for sharing.

This feeling is not confined to villages or small towns. In a big city neighborhood or a suburban street, wherever people come together with their neighbors to weep over sad events or dance and sing and celebrate the happy ones, to help each other in times of need and to share resources, or even just to smile and comment on the weather as they go about their daily tasks, community exists.

I think there are many factors which go to make up this community experience which we find so satisfying to the spirit. One, of course, is that we are basically communal animals. Just like our closest cousins, the chimpanzees, we naturally band together. Another is our sense of identification, whether by birth, by history, by affection—or simply by intent—with the locality. A further vital factor seems to be the physical layout of the buildings and their connecting roads, lanes and pathways. This is something else which Christopher Alexander stresses.[3] There are certain patterns of structure which invite human interaction and others which inhibit it, and town planners often get it wrong. One of the saddest side effects of the slum clearance initiatives of the mid-twentieth century was the destruction of the delicate social fabric which existed in inner city neighborhoods. The architecture of those shabby old tenements in London or New York or those crowded back street workers' cottages of inner city Sydney lent itself to close and frequent connections between people in a way that the newly created concrete tower blocks could never replicate. People were not only removed from their homes and neighborhoods, their links to their communities and landscapes were destroyed as thoughtlessly as a broom crashes through a spider's web. It is no accident that those former slums which were renovated rather than demolished and still retain a semblance of their original layout are often so attractive. They are human-scale places, built for foot traffic and eye-level interaction. They feel communal. So, instinctively, we feel good in them.

With the movement of people out to farther and farther-flung suburbs in search of cheap housing and clean air, came all the problems of isolation, lack of services and the absence of any sense of living community. For I believe that the main factor that makes a locality into a real community is whether or not the people who live there also shop there, eat and drink there, play there, educate themselves and their children there, use all the services which that locality provides and create whatever is missing or needed.

Living in a rural village is not, by itself, a guarantee of this community feeling, for these days, not all villages function as organic communities. Some, unfortunately, have become either dormitories for nearby cities— fancier places for the well-off to live their city lifestyles in—or summer theme parks for tourists. Remoteness from the city can sometimes guarantee the preservation of local community in rural areas. But without that remoteness, the existence of a sense of community is either a matter of luck or the result of someone's determination to save it—or to create it. And it is to this latter phenomenon that I wish briefly to turn, now.

All over the globe, new communities are being created. Co-housing schemes, community development schemes, intentional communities, community gardens in the cities, carpooling—there is no end to the creativity that is emerging. Even as our awareness of our planetary oneness grows, another awareness grows with it, a realization that the globalization of trade is killing off local economies, and with it, the sense of kinship. The

61

saying, "Think globally—Act locally" has been around a while, but it has taken us all this time to soak in its full meaning. "Think globally" has become an urgent imperative, if we are to conserve and protect the limited resources of our planet, but the more global our awareness becomes, the more we realize the importance of diversity, of preserving and restoring the small and the local, of protecting the peasant economies which underpin so many human cultures, and of resisting the imperialism of transnational corporations. "Act locally" means really living where you live and being in a reciprocal relationship with the people in your own locality. It is amazing just how many ways there are to act locally, once you start looking around you.

The other morning, for example, I did two hours counseling, and in return I am getting a new piece of garden furniture. Yesterday I swapped vegetables for fresh eggs. A friend of mine trades foot massage for firewood. Barter is alive and well here and I love it.

However, since it is not always easy to find just the right "fit"—the folks who have what you want may not want what you offer—ways have been found to widen the possibilities. One of the initiatives which has grown from this basic idea is LETS.

For those who have not heard of it, let me explain. LETS (Local Exchange Trading System) is a simple idea which is gaining in popularity worldwide. It enables people to exchange goods and services in just the same way money does, and yet has none of the drawbacks of money, since LETS currency cannot be borrowed or lent and it diminishes, rather than increases, when hoarded.

Last November, our local LETS group put on a fair. I had a stall, packed with goods to sell, some bric-a-brac I no longer wanted, copies of my books, cookies I had baked, little trays of sushi I had made—a whole jumble of things. I sold the lot. And I came home with candles, aromatherapy oils, some handmade Christmas decorations—and a credit balance on my statement. But no money changed hands. I did not even take my purse. I met old friends, and made some new ones. It was a wonderful day.

LETS is just like barter, only much bigger. A LETS scheme can have hundreds—or even thousands—of members trading. The only requirement is that a record of each transaction is made and given to a central administrative body, which keeps records and issues statements to members showing their credit or debit balances.

There is something about this form of trading which I find particularly satisfying. I am not sure what it is. Partly, I suppose, it reinforces a sense of belonging. Money is anonymous. But LETS currency I can only earn or spend within a fifty-mile radius of my home. So there is a certain feeling of specialness about it. Of exclusivity. A sense of "us." The echo, perhaps, of a long ago tribal past.

There is a feeling, too, that one's own possibilities for contribution to the community are somehow wider with LETS than they are with money. When you join a LETS network, you are encouraged to think about all the skills you have. Skills which you may never have thought to offer to anyone else. Skills you would never have dared to try and put a monetary price on. Even though you may have no trade qualifications, for instance, you may have a great talent for DIY projects. A member down the road, who is all thumbs, but could never afford to employ a builder to help him put up his shed, may be delighted to pay you for your time in LETS currency. And you might use that amount to stock up on the organic tomatoes grown by another member, instead of buying the ones at the supermarket, which have been trucked in from several hundred miles away. The tomato grower, who has more tomatoes than her family can use and has already given lots away to her friends and relations, is delighted to get paid for her surplus, and spends the resulting currency on some handmade notepaper which another member has been experimenting with. And so it spreads and grows. People get to know each other. Friendships blossom.

The same principle operates in the system known as Time Dollars, except that what is exchanged for Time Dollars is, as the name suggests, some form of service, from weeding the yard to walking the dog, rather than goods, whereas LETS covers both.

There are about two hundred Time Dollar Exchanges across the U.S. and internationally, ranging in size from dozens to thousands of members. In many ways, time dollars are simpler than regular money, but their implications for social change and community rebirth are enormous. In New York City, women have joined forces to create a skills bank called Womanshare. In inner-city St. Louis, Missouri, Time Dollars have been integrated with the social service delivery system to raise self-esteem and build community.

Yes, I believe that deep down, each of us, even the most introverted, craves a sense of belonging, of being part of a tribe. So I see one of my tasks, as an elderwoman, to be fostering a sense of community through supporting and helping to popularize these simple grassroots alternatives to the creeping globalization—and dehumanization—of our economy. This is one of the many ways in which I work to keep alive the wholesome values of my grandmother's life and bring them into resonance with my own twenty-first century world.

It always delights me to hear of ways in which people have created a community or preserved a failing one. A friend of mine reports that the people in her local area have begun the practice of having a communal meal, once a week, a potluck to which everyone brings something. She loves it and has made new friends this way. Another friend, who is shy and prefers to avoid crowds, says she would hate that. But she gladly feeds her neighbors' cat and waters their plants every time they go on vacation. The action you take may be a huge one, like starting a drop-in center for local youth or forming a playgroup, or a small one, like buying what you need at the local store instead of driving to the nearest shopping mall, carpooling, picking up litter, saying good morning to the folks who pass by with their dogs, welcoming newcomers or attending Neighborhood Watch meetings. But anything you do to foster community is a worthwhile action. We humans need each other and our communities. Like John Donne said back in 1624,

> *No man is an Island, entire of itself;*
> *every man is a piece of the Continent,*
> *a part of the main … .*

So if we let our communities die, part of us dies with them. If we work to revive them or re-create them, we are reviving and re-creating a missing part of ourselves as well. It is a worthy task, and one in which the elderwoman has a vital role to play—at every level.

As she does so, she is demonstrating two further principles which we can now add to our list. They are the principles of comfort and connectedness.

Only if she feels a sense of belonging, relates to the landscape and derives comfort from her surroundings can she connect with her community in a meaningful way. And only by some form of connection to the people around her can she feel fully at home and comfortable. Thus, comfort and connectedness are essential to each other.

simplicity • *deep vision* • *compassion* • *non-attachment* • *Earth-centeredness*
• *comfort* • *connectedness* •

As elders, when we feel comfortable and connected, the impulse towards service invariably arises in us in some form. And when we act upon that, we are in true reciprocal relationship with the community in which we live. Whether the service we perform is as active and obvious as running for mayor or as quiet and unobtrusive as running an errand for a neighbor or praying for the sick of the local parish, it is still service, and all forms of service are equally valuable. It is the quality which matters.

Neither does the service we offer necessarily involve other human beings. Service to the land, the soil, to plants and trees and the landscape around us is equally important. So is service to other non-human creatures. It is to these we turn next.

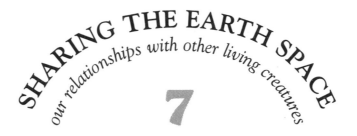

SHARING THE EARTH SPACE
our relationships with other living creatures
7

I RECENTLY re-read (for the umpteenth time) J. Allen Boone's beautiful 1954 classic, *Kinship With All Life*.[1] In it, he tells the story of his apprenticeship to a German Shepherd dog, and how, once he became humble enough to dispense with the mental categories of "man" and "dog," let go of his preconceptions, and approach the project with a receptive mind, a whole new world opened for him. It is a wonderful story. But how many of us would have thought to apprentice ourselves to a dog?

We humans are such an arrogant species that we have even forgotten how closely related we are to all the other creatures who share our Earth, let alone how much all these other beings could teach us, if we listened.

My mother told me that my first non-human teacher was a dog called Patch, who helped my early efforts to walk upright by leading me patiently up and down the garden path with my hand in his mouth. I wish I could remember him. Unfortunately, I don't. However, I do remember several other key teachers who have reached across the species gap to touch my life and change my way of seeing.

One of the most memorable was a teacher I met one summer, quite unexpectedly, in the mountains of south-eastern Australia. I shall always remember our first encounter.

It was a hot, still day; a day of heat haze and blue sky, of eucalyptus scent and the shrilling of cicadas. Inside the cabin, I was eating a solitary lunch and reading a book, glad to be in the shade.

In that valley, summer breezes often begin around midday, bringing cooler afternoons. So when I heard something rustle outside, I looked hopefully out at the peach tree, expecting to see its leaves fluttering. To my surprise they were motionless. Even as I stared, the rustling happened again. Intrigued, I put down my half-eaten sandwich and crossed to the door.

Outside, all was still. No breeze. Just the shimmer of heat on the brick paving. There was another rustle, right by my feet. Then I saw him—a full-sized snake, slithering away towards the bookcase.

I screamed, and leaped outside.

Then, dismayed, I realized my predicament. Inside my cabin, was an Australian brown snake, one of the world's most seriously venomous reptiles. And here was I, on the porch.

I peered in gingerly. "Excuse me," I said. "This is backwards. It is you who are supposed to be out here, not me. Would you mind changing places? Please?"

He took his time, made a full circuit of the cabin, examining everything, his tongue flicking—under the table where a few moments ago I had innocently sat reading my book, under the wood stove, under the dresser. "Oh please," I pleaded, "Don't go in the bedroom." I had no idea what I would do if he decided to hide under the bed and stay there. But he didn't. After a full inspection of the room, he poured himself elegantly out of the door, turned, and disappeared under the cabin.

I sat down, trembling.

Was this how it must have been, I wondered, for Cave Woman? And what of Cave Man, hunting in his bare feet on the forest path, knowing he was potentially both predator and prey and every rustle could be a hungry tiger?

Our tigers are paper tigers nowadays—the only predators the profiteers, hungry for our dollar. We have only ourselves and each other to fear, and our own fearsome creations.

Our modern fears rarely shock us awake into the sudden awareness of mortal danger and thereby into the fullness of the present moment. Rather than powering us for that leap to safety or solution, they send us scrabbling for the remote among the sofa cushions and slipping into a virtual world, suspending our minds, till they are neither weary nor wakeful, merely dulled.

Even in that TV-less cabin, with all the mountain scenery to savor, it was still easy to drift away into those endless rehearsals for the future and rehashings of the past that preoccupy the ever restless mind.

So although I knew he was there, living under my floorboards, half a leg length away, I still forgot the snake. And every time he reappeared, the sight of him shocked me awake again.

One day he was curled up near the outdoor shower. Another time he crossed beneath me as I stood on the stepladder. He had a favorite dozing spot under the apricot tree, and I usually looked for him there. Nevertheless, one morning I forgot, and almost stepped on him. He reared up, and once again my feet left the ground in a hurry. As before, our sudden meeting left me trembling. But as I felt into the trembling, I knew that it was not only fear. There was also an exhilaration—a strange feeling of rightness—as though I were sharing some deep and primeval experience with those ancient, cave-dwelling ancestors.

I began to feel gratitude—almost affection—for this deadly teacher in the grass, with his silent, repeated message. Wake up. Stay awake. Stay in the moment. Stay in your body. Feel your aliveness. Every step you take, take it with awareness. Any moment, you may die. Life is precious, amazing, an adventure.

I nicknamed him Mr. Slitheroe. Whenever I walked outside, I would stamp my foot and call out to him, warning him of my presence, so we could both maintain our necessary distance. I made up a song about him, and I sang it to him as I pottered in the garden.

My partner had been away for several weeks. On his return I told him of the new neighbor below us.

"What do you think we should do about it?" he asked.

"Nothing," I heard myself answer. "Mr. Slitheroe is my Zen master. Every time I forget to live in the moment, he calls me back to awareness with a jolt. I know it sounds weird, but I actually like having him here. I would miss him now. Can you understand that?"

He understood.

Our human neighbors were less understanding.

"You'd be better off hitting him over the head," said one.

"The only good snake," said another, in that laconic way Australians talk, "Is a dead snake."

"You're being irresponsible," said a third.

But leave him we did.

As the days grew shorter and the sun lost its fierceness, he left, migrating to who knows where for the cooler, wetter times. We left too.

I knew that the following summer, someone else would be living in the cabin, picking apricots from the tree, eating their lunch at the table. I wondered if one day they would hear a mysterious rustle or see a sudden movement in the grass. And if that happened, I wondered what those people would do. They may not share my bizarre notion that it can be strangely useful to live a whole summer with a snake-shaped Zen master under the floorboards. However, I knew that I could not alter their destiny, nor Mr. Slitheroe's. We always have to trust that others will make whatever choice is best for them. Including snakes. Whether consciously or otherwise, we each follow the path that is right for us, with all its twists and turns.

If I had killed that slim brown creature who chose to live with us that summer, I would have had another set of feelings to deal with, a different lesson, but perhaps equally valuable. D. H. Lawrence wrote about that experience in his wonderful poem, *Snake*.[2] The hasty, automatic reaction, the guilt that followed his recognition of the impulse to destroy the snake who came to drink at his water trough.

The whole issue of our predatory nature and the killing of other creatures is a thorny one. I am a vegetarian, but I have no quarrel with those who would kill an animal to eat it. We are omnivorous mammals, after all, and meat has long been part of our diet. One of my two reasons for being a vegetarian is a personal one, which is that the killing of other creatures is so painful for me that I cannot do it. Since I cannot do it, it feels morally wrong to turn my back and expect others to do it for me. My simple guideline is that whatever I would have no qualms about removing from its environment myself, I permit myself to eat. Since I can easily pull a carrot or cut a cabbage, or even pluck an oyster off a rock, these I can eat. I could not bring myself to blast a bird out of the sky, to hook a struggling fish out of the water or to plunge a lobster into a boiling vat, so these I refuse to eat. People less squeamish than me can go hunting, and happily devour the flesh of their kill. I have no problem with this. Neither do I have problems with people who can stand, unflinching, in an abattoir, and go home to a blood-red steak. My judgment is reserved for those who recoil in horror at the thought of such a scene and yet can buy pieces of a dead animal wrapped in plastic from the supermarket and draw some sort of mental curtain over the thought of that animal's slaughter. To me, each time we do something like that, we lose awareness. We lose aliveness. We step into the dull, hypnotized world of moral unconsciousness.

My second reason for being a vegetarian is an ideological one, based on the current size of the human population. I believe more people would be able to eat if we all ate low on the food chain. Millions of acres now devoted to cattle grazing or to fodder crops so that the lucky few can eat meat could be used to grow food for the many who now go to bed hungry.

Since I realize that human beings are biologically adapted to eating a varied diet which includes meat as well as all the other things, I have never claimed that meat-eating is less "natural" than vegetarianism. Nevertheless, I do maintain that meat-eating removed from the context of hunting, where hunter and hunted are in relationship, to the context of the modern supermarket, where one is free to claim an animal's body while having no relationship with—or even conscious awareness of—the animal who once lived in it, is unnatural, alienating and destructive of the soul.

When we talk about our relationship with other species, we risk falling into another trap which is more subtle—and much more pleasant to discuss—but equally alienating. This is the trap of anthropomorphism, of attributing human thoughts, feelings and attitudes to other creatures. All those who have lived closely with an animal, be it dog, cat, horse or some other creature, will have been aware of that animal's individual personality, its likes and dislikes, its foibles and phobias and wide range of moods and emotions.

But just because these are recognizable, it does not mean that we fully understand them. In our partial understanding, we have developed the habit of patronizing other species rather than fully respecting and honoring their otherness.

Through our scientific knowledge of that amazing organ, the cerebral cortex, which has given human beings the capacity for abstract thought, a rarely questioned assumption has arisen. This is the assumption that evolution operates rather like an automobile factory, with each year's model being superior in all ways to the previous model. So a starfish is superior to, or "better than," a one-celled organism; a lizard is "better than" a starfish; a rabbit is "better than" a lizard; a monkey is "better than" a rabbit; and a human being is "better than" a monkey—or anything else.

Even with respect to cars this reasoning is not really valid. While today's fast, sleek machine is speedier and more maneuverable than Henry Ford's early models, it is also trickier to repair, uses up more resources in its manufacture, running and repair, dents more easily and causes more accidents. So superiority always depends on what particular factors we are measuring. When it comes to comparing people with each other, we know that it is invalid to make general comparisons. Certainly I can say, from looking at our golf handicaps, that I am a better golfer than you. You, who have won six prizes for cake decorating, can rightly claim to be better at frosting cakes than I am. You are taller, I am fairer, you can hold a tune better than I can, I can run faster... and so on. But neither of us is a superior being. As human beings, we consider ourselves equal.

So I believe that the same thing applies to other creatures. In a game of Scrabble, I would beat a seal every time. But in a swimming contest, the seal would leave me far behind. I am more computer literate than a dolphin or a bat, but my sonar navigation skills are virtually zero. Human beings are less co-operative than bees, less faithful than swans, and most of us are far less stoical than the male emperor penguin who spends the entire Antarctic winter standing in one spot with an egg resting on his feet, with his mate away at sea and blizzards swirling around him.

We are not, as is generally assumed, the end point of evolution. Evolution is more in the shape of a mighty tree, with main branches and minor branches and twigs We are simply one of the farthest twigs from the trunk, that's all.

This does not mean that we have no right to kill other creatures for our own survival. Forms of life have been swallowing other forms of life since Day One—or, more correctly, since a certain day, around fifteen billion years after the Big Bang. That was the day—roughly one billion years ago—when, after three billion years or so of cells minding their own business and living on each other's waste products, a mutation led to the first swallowing of one live one-celled organism by another. And life has fed on life ever since, putting us here, now, at the top of the food chain.[3]

However, being on top of the food chain means only that we are on top of the food chain. It does not give us the moral right to claim any kind of overall superiority. Nor, since we are conscious animals and aware of our actions, does it give us the right to exploit other forms of life heedlessly. The problem, I believe, is in the fact that we humans destroy other creatures not simply for our basic food needs, but for sport, for fun, for convenience, and as a side effect of our profligate way of life.

Apart from the chosen creatures who share our homes as "pets," the ones we enslave as commodities, to eat, experiment upon or use as spare body parts, the opportunistic creatures who colonize our houses, bodies and gardens against our will and with whom we do constant battle, such as rats, fleas, lice, flies, dust mites and garden "pests," our culture seems to view the function of all the others—the ones who live in the wild or in zoos—as the entertainment of humans. Now that we have succeeded in removing ourselves from the dangers of predators, nature has become pretty wallpaper instead of being the matrix of our lives—something to drive around in on Sundays or watch documentaries about from our armchairs.

For me, part of living lightly—especially now, in my elderwoman years—has been the deliberate attempt to re-insert myself into that matrix. One way of doing that is to examine these fundamental issues about how we relate to non-human creatures and to change our thinking about them. In trying to let go of my old stereotyped ways of seeing other creatures and relating to them, I find myself learning unexpected lessons, as I did in my relationship with Mr. Slitheroe. Not only that, but life becomes suddenly richer, deeper, more meaningful.

We have co-evolved with other life-forms. Our bodies are made from the same substances. Our minds have been shaped by interaction with them since the very beginnings of humanity. We are inextricably related. It is not "us" and "them"; it is a huge, universal "we."

In the Native American and the Australian aboriginal cultures, and in some other cultures, this connection is not only honored but taken a step further by the whole concept of totems. The totemic relationship between a group of humans and a particular species of animal is one of a special belonging—a mystical and spiritual bonding.

You may have found this chapter controversial, disturbing, or even irrelevant. I have devoted space to this issue, however, because I have the sense that in our contemporary, Western culture, women generally tend to be more sensitive to the relationship of humans with other creatures than men are. Certainly there have been times in our history when this natural affinity has been strongly disapproved of. During the burning times, for example, when it was generally believed that a witch could change shape at will and become an animal, women could lose their lives for talking in a friendly way to animals, keeping a cat, raising a young animal such as a lamb or even having mice in the house.[4] Traditionally, the witch in pictures is always accompanied by her familiar—usually a cat. All this would seem to suggest a general recognition, throughout history, of women's special relationship with other creatures.

This is why I believe that out of all human beings, the elderwoman is more likely than anyone else on Earth to understand, fully, the changes that need to happen in human thinking for us to be able to come into balance with what Native Americans call "all our relations." In other words, all the other creatures of Earth. I believe she has a better grasp of this than most other people, firstly because she is a woman, secondly because she is a woman of maturity. She is a woman with time to think and to ponder on some of the big philosophical and ethical questions in her culture. Thirdly, as we take up our positions as elderwomen we become aware of the sacred trust we have inherited as the primary keepers of Earth wisdom. Our sacred kinship with the rest of Earth's creatures goes back a very long way indeed.

The change which is needed is for human beings to let go of exploitative and anthropomorphic attitudes to other creatures, substituting feelings of love, admiration and—above all—respect. As elderwomen, we must lead the way.

Among our ranks there are many, I know, whose energy goes directly into improving the lot of other species. For example, when I was a young woman, preoccupied with fashion, beauty and sex, one cultural icon of those times was a voluptuous young film actress with a sexy pout—Brigitte Bardot. Who would have thought, back then, that this same woman, in the third phase of her life, would once more become an icon, but in a very different way. Her tireless devotion to the cause of animal rights made her an elderwoman to be reckoned with.

One word of warning. If any of us should decide to take direct action on animal rights issues, it behooves us to proceed with caution. Well-meaning "rescue" operations by sentimental animal rights activists have been known to wreak environmental havoc by unwittingly unleashing new, exotic predators on vulnerable species of indigenous animals. The ecosystem is a delicate and intricate web. The greatest service we can do it is to respect its complexity. Our main contribution may simply be to re-think this whole issue of relationship between humans and the non-human world and to make our opinions quietly known, as I am doing here.

Back in 1966, in his now-famous paper presented to the American Association for the Advancement of Science, historian Lyn White Jr. suggested that our religion has a lot to answer for in terms of our destruction of the environment. White said that he believed our arrogant exploitation of the natural world would continue until we rejected the misinterpretation of the Bible that made us believe nature has no existence except to serve us.

> *Since the roots of our trouble are so largely religious, the*
> *remedy must also be essentially religious, whether we call it*
> *that or not. We must re-think and refeel our destiny.*[5]

He was speaking about precisely the change in thinking that I have been discussing in this chapter. We need to move away from anthropocentric (human-centered) thinking, in the same way that we had to move away from our former belief that the sun revolved around the Earth. Nothing will change until we do. I believe that the principle we need to call upon in relation to other creatures, as well as other human beings, is the principle of respect. It is one I hope every elderwoman will honor. It therefore becomes the eighth principle on our growing list.

simplicity • deep vision • compassion • non-attachment • Earth-centeredness •
• comfort • connectedness • respect •

Every day at Monkey Mia, on the west coast of Australia, wild dolphins swim to the shore to greet humans. If you stand there quietly, in the shallows, and wait patiently, they will come. I shall never forget the first time I watched a dolphin approach. She swam slowly in front of the row of people, like a general inspecting a parade. Turned on her side, one eye out of the water, she stared up at them, fixing them with her gaze. Excited, I watched her swim towards me, along the row, imagining how our eyes would meet and some magical, New Age-type communion of souls would take place.

Wrong. It was not at all like I had imagined. I can see it now, that dark, intense, penetrating eye meeting mine. But instead of a feeling of connection, I was suddenly overwhelmed by the recognition of our utter and complete difference. And what grew and swelled in me in that moment was a feeling I have never lost. It was the feeling of profound respect. She was forever a dolphin, from the sea world. I was forever a woman, from the land world. Our worlds could never merge, they could only meet at this amazing, respectful edge. I don't know if the same was true for her, but for me, the existence of that edge—that very otherness of hers—has made my whole world ten times more beautiful. It was one of the most precious gifts I have ever been given.

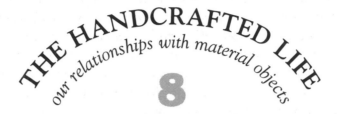

THE HANDCRAFTED LIFE
our relationships with material objects

8

THOUGH I HAVE not seen them for fifty years, I can still clearly remember my grandmother's best bone china cups with the rose motif, and the delicate little saucers they sat on. There were small and large plates to match, various tureens and serving dishes, a teapot, two jugs and a gravy boat. How many years she had owned that set, I have no idea. It may well have been a wedding present. It was the only "good" china she ever had. Most days, she used the half dozen chunky, blue and white Cornish plates and bowls and the plain white cups from the kitchen dresser. But on special occasions or when visitors came, the rosebud things were taken out and proudly used, then stacked away again in the old oak sideboard in the dining-room.

As a child, I always preferred the kitchen china. The other lot, beautiful though it was, seemed too precious, too fragile, too insubstantial to relax with. I decided that when I grew up I would never keep beauty for special occasions. And unlike so many of the women of my grandmother's generation and my mother's, I knew I would never own one of those glass-fronted cabinets in which you keep things which are merely to look at or things too precious for everyday use. I kept both promises.

But that is just me. Each of us has her own relationship with the material objects around her, and each relationship is different.

Nevertheless, as we move into elderhood, there are certain questions common to many of us. This is a time of stocktaking. Do we still need and use all the things we have accumulated during our lifetimes or would it be a good idea to start gradually letting go of them now ? Fine it may be to have cupboards and drawers packed with things we no longer use, but what of the massive sort-out that will be needed when we die? I know of one elderly woman who spent weeks going through her entire house and color-coding everything she owned with adhesive dots so that when she died, everyone would know exactly who was supposed to have what. ("A control freak to the end" was one relative's response!)

There is another question, however, that many of us forget to ask. Do we actually *like* all the things we have?

Over recent years, I have been steadily weeding out plastic wherever I can and replacing it, where necessary, with other materials that I find more aesthetically pleasing. This is a purely idiosyncratic choice, but I derive enormous satisfaction from it. It seems to have some symbolic connection with my increasing need for authenticity at an inner level. Fortunately, my partner is quite tolerant of this process and does not complain when he searches for some particular container and suddenly finds another in its place, especially as he knows I most likely bought it in the thrift store and took the original back there as a donation.

So as we move into our third age, some of us start looking critically at our furniture, our clothing, our possessions of all kinds, and re-assessing their significance to us. It is the time for re-appraisal and—unless we live alone—for re-negotiating such matters with those who share our living space. For this is a stage of our lives when many of us feel the need to ensure that the our home environments express who we are, that anything superfluous or inappropriate is discarded and anything ugly replaced by something beautiful.

Simplifying our lives, which many of us now want to do, is not always easy, however. There are many choices to make: what to keep, what to give away—and to whom—what to throw out. We hear a lot about the importance of the "3 Rs"—repairing, re-using and recycling—but often this is easier said than done. Unless we can do them ourselves, repairs, in this throw-away society, are so expensive as to be almost a luxury. Neighborhood recycling programs rarely keep up with demand and the once traditional re-use of many things—like bottles—has now been swept away by some idiotic health regulation or another.

The more I think about my grandmother's life, the more I realize how full it was of simple, natural hand-crafted and organic things which nowadays would be up-market items, and how lucky she was not to have to bother with so many choices. And she had very little packaging to worry about either.

She wore natural fiber clothing because that is the only sort there was, back then.

She did not have to worry about recycling milk bottles, as the milkman ladled the milk from his churn directly into her big kitchen jugs, which she then covered with natty little hand-crocheted covers, edged with clicketty-clacketty blue beads and put in the larder to keep cool (she never owned a refrigerator). She ate vegetables and fruit in season because they were the only ones available. And they were organically grown and very fresh because she grew most of them herself, in her back garden, hand-weeding them, trapping the slugs with little saucers of beer and picking the caterpillars off the cabbage. The baker's and milkman's horses, if she was lucky, delivered extremely natural fertilizer to a spot right near her front gate, from whence she bore it triumphantly into the garden and on to the compost heap on a shovel while it was still steaming.

Being a dressmaker by trade, my grandmother knew a lot about cloth, so she made quality clothes for us all. In the kitchen, her culinary skills were legendary. All my great-aunts and uncles had their special skills, too, from millinery through winemaking to carpentry. By the time I was ten, I had the belief firmly ingrained in me that homemade things were always of a far superior quality to anything you could buy in a store. I can still hear the echoes of family voices. "Store-bought jelly—oh that's just rubbish. All pips and no flavor." (Well actually, that is not quite accurate. Since we are English, they would no doubt have called it "jam.")

So there was a set of simple rules to follow, back then, for leading the good life. Creating that same good life is not nearly as easy nowadays. We all have so much more knowledge and so many more injunctions rattling around in our heads. If I need a sweater, for example, should I go for natural fiber or synthetic, bearing in mind that the synthetic one (or so my friend Parvati says) might weaken my energy field? If I choose synthetic, do I spend the extra money on Eco Fleece, made from recycled plastic bottles, or the cheaper one which was made from new materials—and were they both made with the same cheap, exploited Asian labor anyway? (In which case I shall either have to pretend I didn't notice or feel guilty and not tell my politically-correct friend Daphne, who would almost certainly do her certain little sniff of mute disapproval.) If I choose natural fiber, do I save up and buy a very expensive, locally made, natural-color wool one, in order to feel good about supporting the sheep farmers and the local craftspeople (and so I'm able to tell Daphne), or a not so expensive wool one dyed with synthetic dyes and, as Daphne would be sure to remind me, brought from miles away using fossil fuels? Do I knit my own—which these days can be an expensive option because fewer people are doing it? (What if I hate knitting?) And how do I feel about wool anyway? Do I worry about overgrazing and the use of organophosphates in sheep dip? What about cotton? Organic cotton is very expensive, and non-organic cotton, I once heard Daphne say, is environmentally polluting. Do I avoid the whole problem by going to the thrift store and buying a secondhand one which has that certain I've-been-in-the-back-of-somebody's-closet-for-years smell clinging to it? (You know the smell I mean, don't you? It is the smell of the thousand stories which still cling persistently to the unwanted garments of their former owners even though those nice volunteer ladies have done their best to wash them off.)

I realize, as I think about all these painful choices, and how hard I have to work to have a simple life like my grandmother's, that there is a beautiful irony about all this. Grandma's life may sound exemplary, but in fact she did what she did as naturally and unquestioningly as the hard-working woodpecker I encountered on yesterday's walk. She lived in a world of simple, natural, handcrafted things and she believed that it was a good world to live in, but beyond that, it took very little mental effort on her part to live that way. She knew no other life, and she died half a century ago. What if she had lived in the year 2000 and something, with a supermarket around the corner, bursting with choices, including not only the pippy, flavorless el cheapo jelly (which by now probably has artificial pips as well as artificial flavoring, not to mention genetically modified something or other) but the best gourmet delicacies from around the world? Had there been money in her purse, she would most likely have filled up her trolley as mindlessly as the next person. If Grandma had access to the sort of shopping malls that I do, she would probably have had a ball. She may well have told me that polyester was marvelous because it never wore out, kept its colors and did not need ironing. And if I tried to explain what Parvati told me about the effect of synthetic fabrics on our subtle energy fields, she would have no doubt have shot me an uncomprehending look and said, "Really dear? Well I never," and gone back to watching her favorite soap opera.

The way I deal with all this is to look beneath the surface and see what "the good life" is really about as regards material objects. What are its elements? One of them, I believe, is the delight factor, (more about this in the next chapter) and another important one is the opportunity to use our creativity, our inventiveness, our natural human ability to solve problems innovatively. When it comes to the acquisition of material things—whatever props or costumes we need in our own particular theatre of life—we find that modern life has to a certain extent denied us a lot of these kinds of opportunities. In particular, it has denied us the chance to improvise.

Did you ever go to Girl Scout camp? I did. Off we used to go, every summer, in a truck, sitting on our kitbags, like soldiers. We had those old-fashioned bell tents, shaped like tepees, with a stout pole in the center. No sewn-in floor. Just the grass underneath. With bottoms you could roll up and something called a "sod cloth" (that felt delicious to say when we were eleven). And we used to furnish them. We made racks for our clothes, racks for our shoes, washstands—all out of sticks found in the woods, lashed together with twine. There was a prize for the best invention. I shall never forget the satisfaction of creating something out of those basic raw materials.

At the end of the week, we had a fancy dress parade. But there was a rule that you must bring nothing from home. Costumes must be improvised from whatever could be found. I remember one year I went as a mermaid. My legs were swathed in a sheet and the top half of me was draped with weeds from the river. I can still feel the slap of cold river weeds against my bare skin, and the water trickling down my back.

Improvisation. It is a wonderful use of the brilliant, ingenious, creative human brain. I suppose this experience that I remember so fondly from my childhood camps was the daily situation for our most ancient ancestors. Stones chipped this way, stones chipped that way, each to fit a purpose. Sticks and rocks, shells and bones and animal skins, the raw materials of forest and prairie, that was all they had. And from there, from that point onwards, down the centuries, the continual stream of human inventiveness has brought us all the way to where we are today, surrounded by more gadgets than we know what to do with.

And it is still going on. Leaf through any mail-order catalog. But what is behind this modern proliferation of gadgets and gizmos and whatsits for every conceivable purpose—and a few inconceivable purposes too? What is it that makes people stay out in their garages, tinkering, till bedtime? What is it that drives people to try and build a better mousetrap? Oh sure, there is the promise of making money. But I suspect that, in most cases, the pure desire to create something new is what happens first.

We all have the creative urge, the fascination with producing something that has never been seen before, the love of novelty. Watch any three-year-old. Some of us lose it. Some of us have it so badly discouraged that we let go of it and forget we ever owned it. But it is part of our natural inheritance, and in each of us it is still there somewhere, albeit buried under layers of other stuff like work and making money and paying taxes and watching videos.

Most of the clever things which people invent are actually a by-product of an instinctual process, i.e. the process of adapting our environment to suit our particular needs, habits, lifestyle, etc. Each of us makes the specific adaptations which pertain only to us. Just as reed-warblers build one sort of nest and goldfinches another, and wrens yet another, each individual human creates the unique nest of his or her choosing—one suited to that particular person and no other.

We do this wherever we are. I remember once visiting a jail and inspecting a row of cells where long-term prisoners were housed. Even in this most rigidly controlled, inhospitable and inflexible environment, I could still see the signs of adaptation, of individuality, of inventiveness. Every inmate, with the barest of resources at his disposal, had managed to make some kind of adaptation. Each cell in the row had a slightly different feel to it. Each was customized to suit its inhabitant.

When the slide projector is at the wrong angle and we prop it up on a telephone book, or we find a new use for an old broom handle, sprout lentils in a jar, reach for an old envelope to use as a bookmark, we are using that same set of skills as the Stone Age man shaping his pointed stone knife, and the very same set of skills as the person who invented that latest gizmo in the catalog. The difference between you and me and that inventor is that we did not happen to feel whatever strong need it was that propelled him or her to create that thingummy with which to fill it. If we had, then we would have come up with something just as good. But it was a need in that other person's life, not in ours. We were busy propping up slide projectors and sprouting lentils while he or she was out in the garage sweating over that one.

We get far fewer opportunities than our Stone Age ancestors did to use our natural inventiveness, for we are so much busier than they were. You might have the idea that the people of those prehistoric days were flat out all day just trying to eat and stay alive. In fact, it has been estimated that they spent a lot less time than we do in such basic tasks as obtaining food. They may have spent a couple of hours a day hunting and another couple gathering plant foods, but in our culture it is normal to spend at least eight hours a day earning the money to buy the food, another few hours a week on top of that actually buying it and bringing it home, and it still needs cooking.

It is a sad and crazy fact that with all these modern, "labor-saving" devices and ready-prepared food, people are actually getting busier all the time. The so-called benefits of modern civilization have given us less time to sit back and enjoy ourselves, not more. With no energy or time left to explore the pleasures and challenges of adapting our environment and using our creativity to the full, we pay someone else to do it for us.

So builders build our houses, factory workers make our clothes, nurserymen grow the seeds and bakers bake the bread. The new slide projector has a special foot that slides up and down, ensuring the correct angle. Lentil sprouts are packaged in a little Styrofoam tray, with clear plastic wrap over it. There is less space left for improvisation.

At the same time, the economics of factory production—particularly when cheap overseas labor is used—are gradually pricing out the artist and the artisan. Handcrafted items are often far more expensive than their mass-produced counterparts. But they have a value which goes beyond the monetary. There is a special satisfaction to be derived from well-made objects that have survived long enough to be handed down from previous generations, or are well enough made in our own times to be handed down to the generations which follow. Although I rarely buy "stuff" any more, I do enjoy, from time to time, the opportunity to throw out some functional but ugly item I have made do with for twenty years and replace it with a handmade equivalent from one of our local craftspeople. And this helps to support them, keeps the money in the local community, and helps to keep the craft alive.

Once we "retire," there is time to think about all this, and to redirect our creativity in more satisfying ways. So now is the time to take a look at the objects that surround you and to decide which of them deserve to remain in your life and which need to leave it. (This applies not only to material objects but also to your choice of ways to fill your day, your choice of ways to have fun, your choice of ways to do virtually everything.)

The increasing desire to drop ballast and have fewer things to care for and worry about is often a natural part of the aging process. Therefore many older women find themselves giving possessions away. For others, though, the new found freedom and opportunities for self-expression bring a desire to accumulate or create objects more in keeping with the people they have now become. I have a friend whose house is now so full of oil paintings she has done since she retired that she is running out of places to hang them.

Even for those of us for whom part of the lightening of getting older is a desire to pare down accumulated personal possessions, parting with objects we have used and loved can still be an emotionally difficult task. It helps to remember that eventually we shall have to be parted from everything, so the earlier we start practicing, the easier it might be. The Buddhist goal of non-attachment does not mean that we repress our feeling of connection to objects—or, for that matter to people, places and ideas—but that we simply accept these feelings, say a gentle "yes" to them, yet do not spend time wallowing round in them and making them worse. It is a tricky discipline, but ideally suited to this life stage.

So whether she is choosing things or losing things, or a bit of both, the elderwoman of today, especially if she wants to walk lightly on the Earth, has to spend a lot of time in decision-making. But the end result is something handmade and beautiful, and therefore nourishing to the soul. For when we truly pay attention to each action, each decision, and its implications, and therefore make each of our choices carefully, prayerfully and in full awareness, what we are actually doing is handcrafting our own lives. And a conscious, lovingly handcrafted life is a wondrous and special thing.

Creativity is the principle which the elderwoman calls upon here, of course. So that must now be added to our list. As Clare Cooper Marcus has shown, our houses—and the material objects we place in and around them—are not merely houses and things but mirrors of our inner selves.[1]

They are the screens upon which our ideals and values are projected. So the elderwoman handcrafting her living space, her third age way of living, is like an artist. She uses her creativity to produce something which is not only beautiful and nourishing to her—and often to others too—but rich in symbolic meaning. This "something" which is her pièce de résistance, her major work, her triumph, is not a picture or a pot, a garden, a quilt or a novel—though any or all of these may form a part of it. It is her elderwoman self, created from the raw material of experience, improvised to suit the needs which have arisen in her life, cut and molded to fit her individuality, polished by the passing of years, decorated with her delight. It fits her and it suits her. And no two are ever quite the same.

With the addition of creativity, our list of elderwoman principles has swelled to nine.

• simplicity • deep vision • compassion • non-attachment • Earth-centeredness •
• comfort • connectedness • respect • creativity •

This chapter has foreshadowed a tenth principle, which I shall now go on to speak of in greater detail. This is the principle I call, simply, "delight."

air

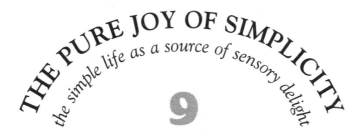

THE PURE JOY OF SIMPLICITY

the simple life as a source of sensory delight

9

LAST SUMMER, at a festival, I took part in a ritual procession. It was late at night, and we were out in the middle of a dark field, with the lights of the campground faint and far away.

Someone had already mapped out the route we were to take, placing unlit flares at intervals along it. As the procession's leaders passed each flare, they set it ablaze. Looking back, we could see the path we had walked, outlined in bright dots of flame.

Life feels a bit like that, to me. We are always walking towards the dark unknown, uncertain of our direction or of the significance of certain special moments. But looking back, we see the connections between them. The patterns they have made.

I recall one such moment from dozens of years ago. It was a beautiful summer afternoon and I was with my partner and our young children, on a hillside near Delphi, in Greece. There was soft, sweet-smelling grass to sit on, and the furry company of bumblebees, busy about their business in the wildflowers. Below us an incomparable view across the Gulf of Corinth and above us the warm and ancient stones of that most magical of places.

The ancient Greeks believed that Delphi was the center of the world, and they marked the spot with a sacred stone, the *omphalos*, or navel of the Earth. It still stands, a squat obelisk, decorated with a delicate tracery of sculpted leaves, guarded from the touch of hands by a stern-faced guard. We had touched it anyway, feather lightly and reverently, accepting as our fate the stern guard's wrath at our disobedience, but knowing that the experience our fingertips had stolen could never be repossessed.

We had walked there from the youth hostel, arriving before the gate was even opened. In the quiet of early morning, we had washed our faces and sipped cool water from the spring, just as the ancient pilgrims did, in purification, before ascending the winding steps of the Sacred Way. We were way ahead of the tour buses, and it was still quiet enough to hear the voice of the Oracle whispering through the pencil pines. When the crowds began to arrive, we were already far above them, sitting in the topmost amphitheater and taking it in turns to run races and do cartwheels for each other's entertainment, watched or maybe even joined in our play by the amused ghosts of long-dead athletes.

By the time the sun was high and the car park full, we had returned to the village for food, and now here we were on the hillside, hungry for our picnic lunch.

Fresh bread, fresh butter, fresh honey and dried figs.

That was all. Fresh, crusty, newly baked bread, white goat's butter, local honey, and the plump brown figs that glistened with the sweetness of last summer's sun. Delicious-tasting spring water to drink.

The utter satisfying simplicity of that meal, assisted by the numinous Delphic energy, reawakened in me a certain feeling from childhood. It was like the feeling that came with the smell of Grandma's bread baking. But I did not realize, until recently, that the path from Grandma's kitchen led to Delphi, and the path from Delphi led directly to here, to now, and to my struggle to articulate exactly what it is that makes the essential difference between being an old woman and being an elderwoman. It has birthed in me this strong dedication I now feel to bringing the elderwoman quality forward, not only into my own life, but into a society which has gone searching for its happiness in all the wrong places and has drawn increasingly desperate blanks. It is a personal voyage of discovery which is also a shared one.

As we have seen, the elderwoman quality derives from certain principles, which we are in the process of exploring. These memories of Delphi illustrate what I have called—for want of a better name—the principle of delight.

The particular kind of delight that I am speaking of is more than just the ordinary delight you feel when something nice comes in the mail. It seems to have more dimensions than that. It is a feeling of fullness and aliveness and ordinary sacredness. Yes, it comes with the smell of baking bread, but it is more than just the delicious smell of baking bread. It is what you get when you combine the smell of the bread with the nutritional value of the wholewheat grains, the shape of the farmhouse loaf, the simplicity and solidity of an old-fashioned bread oven, the coziness of the kitchen, the meditative movement of hands kneading dough and the love that goes into the baking. Add them all up, and the result is a sense of organic naturalness and simplicity and wholeness, which the word "delight" cannot fully describe. But it will have to do, for now, since I can find no better one in our language. It is very similar to what the Japanese call *wabi-sabi*—the principle underlying those things of simple elegance for which the Japanese culture is so famous, such as ikebana (flower arrangement) and the tea ceremony, things of refinement which have yet retained their essential naturalness, their clear lines and rustic character.[1]

A prerequisite for this kind of delight to arise in our lives is quiet attention to the moment, for the *wabi-sabi* quality can only be fully appreciated by a mind which is at once peaceful and yet fully attentive. Another is an underlying attitude of trust and "enoughness"—something I shall be speaking of at greater length in Chapter 11. For when the bread is baked, we cannot savor it unless we rest into the process. To gobble it and rush on to the next activity is to miss the point—and miss out on the delight.

Many years later, visiting Greece again, I searched in vain for the goat's butter and the honey. The wonders of modern marketing had brought in butter from New Zealand and replaced the local honey with a large assortment of those little plastic containers of Kraft spreads. I guess they call it progress, but to me it feels more like theft. The theft of delight.

It made me sad; not only because the quality was lost, but because I know that the kind of food from which that humble picnic on the hillside was made is slowly being replaced, worldwide, by something less nutritious and less beautiful, for food can be beautiful, not only in its taste, but in the way it looks, the way it smells, the way it feels. And another experience, similar to the Delphi picnic, brought that home to me, right in the middle of a very ordinary day.

It happened way back in the days before I had a garden. I belonged to an organic fruit and vegetable co-op. It was at the unfashionable end of a dusty city street. A simple, unglamorous shop, with a cement floor and big wooden benches lined with boxes of produce. Most of the staff were volunteers, who worked in return for generous discounts. It felt good in there. Customers chatted and smiled, weighing out their own produce and jotting down the prices themselves on little pads of scratch paper with stubby pencils attached. There were a few recycled bags. Many people, like me, brought baskets.

This particular morning, I had walked out of the co-op with a full basket and was attaching it to the pack-rack of my bicycle, when suddenly the sheer beauty of that basketful of fruit and vegetables made me stop and stare. It was like a piece of art. The dark green of the chard leaves and the bright yellow of the tiny squash that nestled among them, the earthy promise of the mushrooms, the translucent glow of the apples and carrots, all mixed together in the basket, suddenly took on an aura of beauty that surpassed any painting I had ever seen. Gifts of the field. How utterly beautiful they all looked, sitting there together. A colorful cornucopia of nourishment. Remembering other places I had lived, other ways I had shopped, remembering Styrofoam and shrink-wrap, plastic bags inside plastic bags, I felt suddenly overwhelmed by emotion. It was as though blessings were raining down upon my head. A golden, glowing moment of delight.

I realized in that moment, standing beside my bicycle, that living lightly is not just about being kinder to the Earth and obediently doing the right thing, ecologically. It is about pure pleasure. It is about stopping and noticing and being aware, for it is through that very awareness that the delight begins to flow. It came to me, right then, as I stood there smiling at my fruit and vegetables, that for me to have to buy them at the supermarket would actually be to deprive myself of something wonderful.

Yes, the organically grown produce cost me a little more, that's true. But I did not begrudge a cent of it, for the things I bought were fresh and alive and my buying of them was an act of communion with the soil that bore them and the sun that ripened them. It was, too, a vote of confidence in the people who work that little bit harder in order to preserve the integrity of the soil and let its millions of living organisms do their work as nature intended, free from the threat of destruction by chemicals. I knew that the price I paid was the true price, rather than an artificially low price achieved by the ruthless and exploitative methods of large-scale agribusiness. Furthermore, the fruit and vegetables on sale at the co-op were usually those locally in season. Waiting until the Earth rolled around and conditions brought forth the right crops at the right times helped me to stay in touch with the movement of the Earth and the passage of the days. It seemed to me that so much in our modern lives dislocates this sense of natural rhythm. Growing one's own vegetables, it is easy and automatic to eat seasonally. But if you live in the city, surrounded by a vast selection of food imported from every corner of the globe, the simple joys of seasonality are soon lost. Nothing is special any more. The lazy overabundance of the modern supermarket has an overall deadening effect; a gradual lessening of awareness of the seasonal cycle and a dull boredom with the sameness of plenty.

It may also be bad for our health. In Oriental medicine, there is the notion that the fruits of each season are appropriate nourishment for the body in that particular season. The cool, wet watermelon that we rejoice in on the red hot days of summer, if eaten in winter would chill the bones that call out for the comfort of soup and the warming flush of chilies. It makes sense. Our earliest ancestors lived in this way. It is how our bodies were designed to function.

For thousands of years, our ancestors grew their own food. And for millions of years before that, they foraged for it. Maybe this is why growing one's own food feels so satisfying. It is like a homecoming. It has certainly been one of the chief delights of my life. How good it tastes, my own produce in the cooking pot. Feeding my children on it was like giving them my own milk. Simplicity is not a strange or new concept. It is one of the oldest in existence. It is where we belong. Food we have grown, fruits and vegetables in season, the rhythms of Nature soothe and comfort. Alienated from those rhythms, we wander lost in the artificial world we never intended to make.

So there were many messages for me, folded into that moment outside the co-op, with one hand on my bicycle.

I love those special moments. When I have dozed off into mindlessness, they wake me up again, like alarm clocks, bringing new messages of wisdom. They recall me to aliveness, inviting me into wonderment and into the fullness of living. And they can happen any time. Even in the middle of the shopping. The older I get, the more of those moments I seem to have. It is, I now realize, one of the key benefits of living one's old age the elderwoman way, a benefit I never expected.

It reminds me of the surprise I got when I discovered how physically pleasurable it is to suckle a child. For some strange reason, no one ever tells you that before you become a mother. You hear all about cracked nipples and about how much better a mother's milk is for the baby and it sounds like something you do because it is, well, a good thing to do. Then—once you get past the ouch of the cracked nipple stage—you suddenly discover that it actually feels wonderful to you as well as to the baby.

Likewise, the sheer pleasure of simplicity is seldom mentioned. There are many books written about how we should be kind to the Earth and live in harmony with nature, recycle, compost, and on and on. It is true that if we wish to save the aspects of our planet which so many of us love—the rainforests, the diversity of species, the pure air and clean water and so on—then those of us who live in the West will have to learn to become materially poor again, to embrace a simple life and to give up the wealthy, wasteful lifestyles, which have brought us to the edge of disaster. But so often when that is written or spoken, it sounds like a penance. Like nasty medicine, perhaps, that we must swallow in order to heal ourselves before it is too late. On the contrary, I have discovered, as I have moved further and further into the contemplation and the living of it, that this potion we must drink may not be nasty medicine at all, but rather a precious nectar that we are privileged to sip. The light and simple lifestyle, when we can truly enter into it—when we can stop rushing about and take a moment to appreciate it—begins to reveal itself as one of the most delightful things that a life on Earth has to offer.

This delight is, theoretically, available to us at any stage of our lives. However, the younger and busier we are, the more preoccupied with making a living, raising a family, pursuing careers, establishing a sound financial basis for ourselves and all of that, the harder it is to stand still long enough to discover it. Sure, we may read about this sort of thing. But no matter how much we study and how learned we become, all the accumulated riches of the world's wisdom traditions cannot be more than a dry collection of words and concepts until we have lived that wisdom and felt it echo in our cells, come alive in our bones.

So when we move into the third age, at last we are truly ready for the simple contemplative life. Now we are truly able to understand and practice that lifestyle which before had seemed so unattainable. Now we can move into it as easily as a ripe apple falls from a tree. A life of simple, healthy, sensual living is one perfectly suited to the last third of life, enabling us to savor that life fully, to its very last drop.

• simplicity • deep vision • compassion • non-attachment •
• Earth-centeredness • comfort • connectedness • respect • creativity • delight •

In coming again to simplicity, and in embracing the delight principle, we come full circle to the first comforts of our human experience. The memory of these, though erased from conscious awareness, still lives in there somewhere. In fact, I believe that each one of our moments of sensory delight is only possible because of the moments which have gone before. Perhaps there is no original moment. Perhaps each special experience we recall owes part of its specialness to the fact that we are already alerted to its possibilities by an earlier experience; already programmed by some earlier happening to have our memories jogged. Moments have their ancestors, stretching back into our lives and perhaps beyond them to former lives, who knows? Or maybe, beyond it all, there is some archetypal set of experiences which each soul dimly remembers, brought to life in the re-living. If we are all one consciousness, then the ultimate ancestor of our moments is the common ancestor, the unconscious memory bank which belongs to all and one.

I remember another simple meal which was given to me when I was still a child. Arriving one summer evening, after a long journey, I was brought to the farm where my grandparents were staying. I was groggy with weariness from my journey, but since I had come too late for dinner, I was a little hungry. I remember the tiny attic room they showed me to, the comfy bed, the peace and quiet of the countryside, and the farmer's wife coming in with a tray. On it was a tall glass of milk, still warm from the evening milking and a huge crust of fresh bread, spread with homemade butter—a meal similar to the one at Delphi, all those years later.

That meal still lives with me. I can taste the butter, feel the texture of the bread and the animal warmth of that milk fresh from udder of the cow. It was total simplicity and total bliss.

I suppose, if you think about it, most of our childhood happiness came from simple things. Our first comfort, after all, was the simplicity of the nursing breast and the taste of warm, sweet milk. Probably that was why my glass of cow-warm milk tasted so good that I almost could not drink it, so overwhelmed was I by the taste and smell and feel of it. If every moment has its ancestors, the ancestors of that one were almost certainly the basic and blissful delights of the satisfied infant.

The savoring of simple food is one of the easiest ways to lead ourselves into a deeper sensory awareness and thus to a greater feeling of aliveness. So I would like to end this chapter by introducing you to an exercise which aims to bring the delight of simplicity alive in your own five senses, right here and now, in a very *wabi-sabi* kind of way. You might care to try it. I call it the Raisin Meditation.

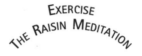

EXERCISE
THE RAISIN MEDITATION

You may find it best to read this exercise through first and then do it, rather than trying to read it and do it at the same time.

I use those plump and rich-brown muscatel raisins that come with the stalks attached, because the flavor is so rich and I love them. But you could use anything—a piece of full-flavored, organically grown apple, for instance, or a strawberry, but only if they are in season. When we eat the fruit which is growing naturally around us, in its own season, it gives fully of itself and seems to nourish us more fully on every level of our being. Dried fruit is fine though. It saves it sweetness for us, long after its growing season is past. Another favorite taste treat of mine is dried mango. I know where to buy the fair-traded ones, so that when I eat them I know that whoever picked and processed this fruit was properly rewarded for his or her labors. And the fact that it comes from far away and therefore cost a lot of energy to bring to my plate means that it is something I only allow myself to indulge in very, very rarely, perhaps on special occasions like Christmas or my birthday.

Whatever you choose for this exercise, make sure it is something you love the taste of.

Place the raisin (or whatever you have chosen to substitute) on a small and pretty plate, in a little basket or on some kind of ceremonial dish or container, which may be anything, a special hanky, a seashell, whatever takes your fancy. This act of choosing a special container is important. It is one of the things which turns an otherwise ordinary act into a ritual. Just as the Japanese use a special teapot for the tea ceremony, or Christians use a chalice and paten for their wine and wafers, our raisin needs its ritual container.

Sit in a quiet, comfortable, undisturbed place, and relax. Allow the busyness of the day to drop away.

Take a little time to explore, inwardly, noticing where there are lingering places of tension in your body. Acknowledge each one and thank your body silently for these attempts to armor you against the problems and difficulties of the outside world. Then gently let each tension go.

Give your mind time to slow down and become quiet. The Buddhist teacher, Thich Nhat Hanh says that when we sit down to meditate, we are a bit like a glass of cloudy apple juice. When you let it sit quietly for a while, it clears. Sit quietly, and gently allow your body to relax and your mind to clear.

When you feel ready, take the raisin from its container and look at it carefully. Notice its shape, color, texture. Visualize it growing—how it developed and ripened in the warmth of the sun. Let yourself feel a sense of appreciation for it, as a gift to you from the sun.

Put the raisin in your mouth and hold it there, exploring it slowly. You may choose to do this with your eyes closed. Feel the saliva coming in as your body prepares to begin the work of absorbing this new food.

Gently break its skin with your teeth and feel the flavor burst upon your senses. Roll it around in your mouth. Chew it slowly, slowly, savoring every movement, every sensation, fully feeling it, concentrating your whole being on the taste, the texture, the experience of eating this one small thing very, very slowly and reverently.

Swallow it only when it has become fully liquefied. Then savor the taste which remains upon your palate, just as a wine taster savors a fine wine. Give thanks once again, to the food itself and the sun which grew it, and to yourself for the opportunity to have this experience.

Before you return to the ordinary world, take a few moments to review your body again and check that the once tense places remain calm and relaxed. Make some gesture, like placing your palms together, or whatever *occurs to you, to signify the closing of your private ritual, and wash, wipe or ritually dust off the container that you used before returning it to the everyday world also.*

Allow yourself time to let the effects of this deceptively simple exercise reach your being at all levels.

And by the way, don't beat yourself up for not eating every meal in that slow and meditative way. Don't burden yourself with good resolutions. This was an exercise, not a prescription. So just put the dish away and get on with your life. Or the next chapter.

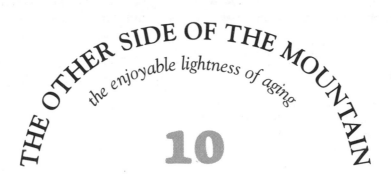

THE OTHER SIDE OF THE MOUNTAIN
the enjoyable lightness of aging

10

THE NEXT principle—the eleventh—is the principle of lightness. Once again, as I search for pictures to illustrated my meanings, I find myself once more in southern Greece, in the place they call Arcadia. It is several decades now, since I traveled through the valley of Arcadia, but my memory of it is as vivid as ever.

Arcadia. The name conjures up visions of nymphs and shepherds frolicking in a lush green landscape, heavy with the fruits of nature.

That was how it felt, too, sitting on that old navy-blue bus as we wound our way round narrow and precipitous bends to the accompaniment of bouncy Greek music on the bus radio—lush and full; life as endless, plentiful adventure.

Arcadia. Fabled valley of the gods and goddesses, countryside rich and full with history, exquisite still in its green and fruitful beauty. I remember it as though it were yesterday, and that feeling of adventure and excitement rises again in me as I hear, in memory, the sound of Greek voices against the rumble of the old engine. I recall how we stopped for three musicians to climb aboard, and how they played their instruments all the way to the next village. I can still see, in my mind's eye, the faded pictures of saints pinned around the edges of the driver's cabin, the dangling beads and good luck charms that kept us all safe as we sped down hills and around corners, and the roadside shrines I was trying hard not to think about too much despite my children's ghoulish cries of "Look Mom, there's where another one went over!"

Somewhere on that journey, climbing high, we crossed the mountainous spine of the Peloponnissos and turned a corner into a different world. Verdant wood and pasture gave way to olive grove and rocky hillside. Wet and lush gave way to dry and sparse. We were on the other side of the mountain. Around Tripolis, oranges grew in the white sunlight, heat bounced off bare stone. And it was that way all the way to the coast, to the turquoise waters of the Argolian Gulf

I used to bleed, back then.

I was like Arcadia, lush and fruitful in my bleeding, my mothering, my womanhood. My sap flowed, just as it did in those green oaks and sycamores that lined the valley, overhung the road, filtering the sunlight.

Somewhere along the way, I reached a peak, half recognized in the busyness of a full life, and traveled for a while along the ridge, just as the road does before it winds down to Tripolis.

The ridge, of course, was menopause, and it lasted quite a while. There was protest in my body as the sap began to leave; protest in my mind as the landscape of my life began to change; turmoil in my heart, assuaged somewhat through the writing and sharing of my own experience. But when I emerged from it, I found that I had turned the corner. I was on the other side of the mountain. And there was a whole new lightness in my being. The hot flashes and night sweats ebbed away, leaving my body quieter, softer, dryer; lighter, as a leaf gets lighter before it falls. My energy returned. Not quite with the same force as before. This energy has a different quality somehow. For one thing, the daily allocation is slightly less. A highly productive morning needs to be followed by a quieter afternoon. I can no longer squander reserves, for if I do, the well is empty for several days afterwards. But there is a wirier, more reliable energy under there which, if it is not abused, remains constant every day, unlike the fluctuations that hormones once dictated.

It is not the endless energy of the child, freely spent and totally renewed by a short nap. It is a slow but steady, even-paced energy, resilient like desert grass.

Something else I realize now, in retrospect, looking back at all my years of motherhood, is that motherhood gave me a feeling of being somehow at the center of things. As though the world revolved around me. Not in a narcissistic way, as though I were the only important person around and needed everyone's attention. We all know people like that and I hope I am not one.

No, I mean central in a cozy sort of way, with a sense of being at the heart of a nest to which everyone came home; fully present as an essential part of the fulcrum around which all our lives revolved. That, too, felt like Arcadia. Nymphs and shepherds in intimate-looking groups, lying around with their limbs touching, like the ones in those old oil paintings.

Nowadays, my children have nests of their own. I am no longer the center of anything except of myself. So the challenge of that has been to re-orient myself to the world in such a way that I don't keep feeling as though something is missing

In my work world, the pattern was similar. Retired, from an organization I helped to create, I found myself no longer at that hub either.

This seems to be the deeper dynamic behind the "empty nest syndrome" and the angst that many feel upon retirement from a career. It is not just that you miss your kids because they have grown up and left, or that you are wondering what to do with your life now that it no longer revolves around the workplace. It is that you have to move out of the feeling of being at the center of things, and the coziness which went with that, and face life from a different place. It takes courage, for this land can be dry, rather than lush and cozy.

Some people remain in denial. They block the feelings with busyness, TV, or any one of a hundred ways that human beings have devised in order not to stay awake to the experience of their own lives. Others look ahead for ways to cope.

The first impulse, quite often, is to try to rewind to an earlier version of the self. But that long-ago self seems two-dimensional now, empty, shallow, a costume for a play whose season is long since over. The old roles, the old selves, they are quite inappropriate for nowadays, even if we could still remember our lines. The selves who stare back at us from the photos of our youth are like characters playing parts for which the scripts are now lost. As Helen Luke points out in *Old Age: Journey into Simplicity*, it is imperative that we do not follow this impulse but turn, instead, towards the true tasks of aging.[1]

At first, as we look in all the old places for inspiration, and do not find it there, there is a sense of disappointment and disillusionment. It is easy to fall into depression, wondering if all the meaning has gone from life and it would be better to die now and be done with it.

This is a key point in our lives. It is at this point that the choice is made, albeit often without fully realizing that we are making a choice. It is from here that two roads lead forward. One is the road of resignation. The road that leads to nowhere except a weary, dreary waiting room in which we try to keep ourselves occupied while we wait the call of death. The other is the way of the elderwoman. This is the path that leads at first to the desert, for it is in the desert that we shall discover our true strength.

The desert, when one first encounters it, seems bare. The very word "desert" implies barrenness, emptiness, isolation. But for anyone who walks in the desert with fully open eyes there is a revelation waiting. The desert teems with life. Tough, resilient, wiry life, dry and enduring in the heat of day and cold of night, conserving the rain that falls so rarely, living, relating, being, in the full glare of the sun and the starry desert dark.

The elderwoman's life, on the far side of menopause, is like the desert. Stark, real, beautiful and full of a different kind of life. This is not the ascetic life of a spirit that denies the body and yearns to transcend it. Far from it. This is the life of a spirit that drops ever more deeply into the body, hangs in with the body as it dries and ages and withers, feels it from the inside, marvels at it as it goes through its stages and the bones creep ever closer to the surface.

There is another image which I would like to share with you. Once, when I lived in a warmer climate than I do now, my garden grew tomatilloes, those little Mexican tomatoes that grow inside a husk. They were everywhere, their vines sprawling lushly all over the place in eager fertility. Thousands of fruit fell to the ground. Some we ate, some we bartered or gave away, some simply lay there and rotted. Eventually, the frosts came, the leaves and stems blackened and fell, and the last of the fruit returned squishily to earth. For a while, the smell of fermentation hung in the air, and then the brown humus reclaimed its own. Winter was upon us and the places where the summer's tomatilloes had flourished were bare again.

One warm day in spring, foraging for carrots, I found the most exquisite little parcel, sitting neatly on the ground. What had once been a tomatillo was now a delicate basket of filigree lace, almost non-existent in its sheer transparency, a perfect basket-shaped skeleton. Inside it, rattling there like so many marbles in a bag, a few dozen seeds. Nothing more. The bare essentials that remained of a tomatillo fruit, a packet of seeds in nature's own presentation pack.

I held it reverently in my hand. It reminded me of the desert, of how the deep basics of life are exposed when the flesh dies and the skeleton bleaches in the sun. It reminded me of myself, as I grow old and let go of all but the hardy, long-lasting essentials. It seemed to me the perfect symbol of the elderwoman.

This is the essence of the grandmother's lightness, the lightness of aging gracefully, of aging fully, and letting the passions of a fully-lived life burn you right through to ash.

Probably, I would feel out of place in Arcadia now. My task is to make my life on the other side of the mountain, among the orange groves; to feel all right as a tomatillo husk lying undiscovered on the earth, far from the cozy center of things; to conserve my resources, as a desert dweller should, and to welcome into my bones that very sun that will one day bleach them white. For when life has fully burned me up, then I can go home satisfied, leaving only my seeds and the faint filigree husk of a memory.

Lightness, then, for an elderwoman, is who she is. It is also how she lives. In the effort to make our footprints upon the Earth as light as possible, and to give back as much as—or more than—we take out, we are respecting this beautiful planet of which we are a part. So let's add lightness, now, to our list of elderwoman principles.

• simplicity • deep vision • compassion • non-attachment •
•Earth-centeredness • comfort • connectedness • respect • creativity •
• delight • lightness •

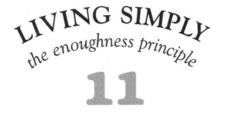

LIVING SIMPLY
the enoughness principle
11

I AM GOING to start this chapter by talking about food again. My friends tease me about being obsessed with food, and I do not deny it. Food is one of the finest pleasures of my life. And since eating is perhaps the best and simplest way to look at our next principle—the one I call "enoughness"— I shall start by reminiscing about a certain meal.

It is more than ten years, now, since that first meal I ate at Daniela's house, but I remember clearly the moment of walking into her dining room.

The large, solid dining table was matched by four substantial-looking chairs upholstered in a plain soft fabric. It all felt spacious, gracious, ample—and yet simple. The table was set with four places, each with one elegant bowl, a matching plate, a cloth napkin, and a pair of delicate black lacquer chopsticks, the Japanese kind with tapered tips. The room seemed to welcome us, embrace us. Soft lamplight twinkled on the surfaces of the bowls and on the smooth lacquer of the chopsticks. The evening suddenly seemed full and rich, and I felt already fed and warmed, just from the beauty of the table and the joy and ease of being with my three companions.

Daniela brought in the food. A platter of lightly steamed vegetables, spread in colorful layers, a covered bowl of brown rice, four plump yellow corn cobs gleaming on a plate, and two small bowls, one holding a creamy, piquant sesame sauce and the other a garnish of fresh cilantro.

Carefully, we measured rice into our bowls and topped it with the vegetables, spooning on the sauce and adding some pungent green cilantro leaves. There was exactly enough to go round. No more, no less. And one corn cob for each of us. We sank teeth into the juicy kernels.

With chopsticks, you tend to focus. These delicate tools can spear a tiny floret of broccoli with precision, can scoop up exactly the right amount of rice for the mouth to deal with in that moment.

Eating like this becomes a meditation. Every mouthful is a festival of awareness. Color, texture, flavor, warmth, juiciness, crunchiness, mushiness. The feel of food in your mouth, the responses of your taste buds, the aroma. Subtleties reveal themselves.

As I recall this dinner at Daniela's and the way the very simplicity and elegance of her proffered meal brought my attention to focus on the food I was eating, I have another memory, this time of the Kripalu Center, in western Massachusetts, where I first went in 1985. There, we ate in silence, men in one half of the dining-hall, women in the other. That was where I first learned the simple discipline of focusing totally on my food, freed from the obligation to communicate, yet not permitted to escape into a book or magazine. It was a way of meditating; of learning to appreciate the nourishment that was entering our bodies and remaining fully conscious in the moment. Yet despite this wonderful opportunity for re-connection with the food I ate, I did not always achieve that one-pointedness. As in any other meditation, the mind easily wanders off, away from the moment, into reverie. And mine often did, during my weeks of living and eating there. It would wander into the past or the future, rehearsing what may be to come or re-hashing what had already been, re-arranging memories to compose a more palatable history, squeezing another drop from pleasures past, or vainly attempting to devise ways of controlling the uncontrollable, unforeseeable time-yet-to-come. In one way, it was a splendid opportunity, a chance to practice the simple enjoyment of food. But in another sense, it was a burden, for it provided me with yet more ways to stumble and fall and to notice and judge and sigh over my own imperfections.

For some reason, that night at Daniela's house, the freedom to talk and be distracted did not take me away from the mellow meditative mood. I ate my food slowly and savored every mouthful, all the while savoring, just as fully, the pleasure of sharing the company. It seemed to me that the magic of the evening arose partly out of the simple elegance for which Daniela is renowned, and partly from the sharing, but mostly out of the exact rightness of the amount of food.

For dessert, there was a plump and juicy orange, complete in its globular wholeness, its integrity of skin and pith, flesh, pip and juice. Segments of flavor that exploded between the teeth.

We sat long at the table, joined in our conversation and laughter, until the evening grew old and the yawns began. A perfect evening, perfectly complete.

It set me wondering about the whole issue of simplicity and what that word really means. Only a week earlier, I had entertained a whole raft of relatives in our tiny cottage. I had cooked all day. Every available pot and pan had been called into service. Every dish and bowl seemed to be needed to accommodate the occasion. Since there was no dining room in the cottage, and the little kitchen table could seat only four people—and that with a severe squeeze—it was a matter of putting all the food out and then inviting people to fill their plates and find a spot to sit, balancing their meals on their laps. There were bodies in all the chairs, on the piano stool, some on the floor and one or two even on the stairs. It was chaotic, yet it was simple and friendly. At their houses, there are tables that can seat a crowd, vast dinner sets that can be taken from cupboards for such occasions, dishwashers to churn through the resultant pile of messy crockery and cutlery. In our little cottage, there was only the small pile of unmatched plates from the thrift store, the little basket of knives, forks and spoons, a few mugs and bowls and other odds and ends. There was only one tiny kitchen bench, one small draining board and one wash-up brush with which to restore the shine to the dishes. But it worked, somehow, We washed up the soup bowls so we could have fruit salad in them. We took turns in the chairs. We made do. Everyone was fed and everyone was happy.

There seem to be so many versions of simplicity. Mine was in the cottage and its limitations, and I gave the occasion as a gift to my extended family members. To them, I gave the experience of making-do in a small space and discovering that it can be done—just as one improvises at a picnic or on a camping trip—and the intimate conviviality of washing the bowls for a second use and squeezing together on the sofa.

It could be that the difference, the way of doing things which is so foreign from their own, the indoor picnic, gave them a chance to be alive and aware instead of living out of habit. For me, to whom life in the cottage was routine, that aliveness came instead from the state of emergency, the need to stretch resources, to ransack the attic for one more bowl or to juggle saucepans and bench space, preparing dinner for fifteen in a kitchen built for two.

For all of us, for the space of one evening, it created the opportunity to be conscious rather than asleep. So, although I gave them food because I love them and wanted to share time with them, I also gave them the gift of my particular version of simplicity.

The cost was in the six bowls of leftovers I tried to cram into our tiny refrigerator that night, monuments to my overestimation. It was also in the tiredness that overwhelmed me when the day was done and the last guest overstayed my limits of coping, and in the bloated stomachs of those who filled their plates again and again out of my overabundance and then had to loosen their belts. It was an abundance that came not just from love but also from the fear of scarcity, the fear of falling short, of not being loved— or loving—enough. It came from the need to compensate; to be seen and appreciated as Demeter, the Earth Mother, eternally giving and nurturing, always needing to be needed. Although we can recognize those needs in ourselves, sometimes it takes a while to outgrow them. In the meantime, we can simply observe them, just as in the Kripalu dining-hall I observed the wanderings of my ever restless mind.

To be sure, there was love in my giving of all that food, but it was in a way the misguided love of a mother who makes her baby fat and leaves him a lifetime legacy of obesity. I gave to my guests the simplicity of a cottage meal, and at the same time I gave myself another in that line of frank portraits that sees me as I am, a mixture of noble and ignoble motives, of light and dark, of persona and of shadow.

In retrospect, as I ponder on these issues of food and feeding and the gift of one's simplicity to another, I can see that there are many ways to do it and many lessons to learn from it. I realize now that the simple perfection of Daniela's meal was that it came in exactly the right amount. The spare elegance of bowl and chopstick was a gift as well. Like the beautiful accoutrements of the Japanese tea ceremony, that elegance served to create an ambience wherein the ordinary can take on the quality of sacredness. For me, the deepest gift of that night was the experience of sufficiency, exquisitely judged. We are so accustomed to helping ourselves from a loaded table and storing the leftovers that we take our platefuls for granted, forking them absentmindedly into our mouths, swallowing them half-chewed, waking from our automatic stupor only when the signal comes, too late, from an already overloaded stomach. On that rare occasion when the amount is right, there is time to chew and to savor, and yet time and space to talk and laugh and share as well. A meal like that becomes a meditation on being alive, in a healthy body, nourishing one's cells with the gifts of the garden and one's soul with the gifts of congenial companionship and an underlying sense of the sacred in all things.

Thinking back, next day, on that simple shared meal at Daniela's, I remember saying to myself "If only our whole lives could be like that."

But they could be, of course. All it takes is full attention to each moment and a willingness to share whatever is presented to us in that moment, knowing that it is exactly right—which, as we all know, is easier said than done. Once in a while, we do get it just right. And the result is magic.

The funny, ironic postscript to this is that when I mentioned to Daniela, the other day, that I was writing about that long-ago meal, she could not remember it. And when I described it she said, "Gosh, I must have been running low on food that day, and scraped up a meal out of what I could find!" I laughed. Like I said, once in a while, we get it right. Even when it happens by accident.

It was a useful accident, as so many accidents are, when you look back at them with elderwoman vision. For that meal at Daniela's house, all those years ago, was perhaps the first time I thought consciously about what I now call the Enoughness Principle.

Why, I wondered, is it often so difficult for us human beings to hold up our hands and say "*enough*!"? Why is it so difficult to refuse a second helping, one more drink, one more chocolate from the box? "I shouldn't really…" we say, glancing sideways at each other, "but… oh what the hell?"

Once, when I ordered the "mild" version of a curry and found it still far too hot for my taste buds, I asked the manager of the curry-house why they put so much chili in. "It started off as a mild dish," he replied, "but as time went on, the customers seemed to want it hotter and hotter, so we just put more and more in to keep them satisfied." The same thing often happens with salt in manufactured foods, and also with sugar.

Chili, salt, sugar, money, profits, growth, gadgets, you-name-it—where is the "*enough*!" master-switch in our brains that tells us when a limit has been reached? The answer is, of course, that there isn't one. At the level of certain bodily systems, like hunger, thirst or sex, there is a satiety point at which the body, like an electric battery, says "That's enough for now, I need to recharge." But that kind of enough is a temporary one. After a certain period of time, known in physiology as the refractory period, desire reasserts itself. There is no automatic switch that says "You now have enough money, enough possessions, enough achievements to last you the rest of your life." We have no inbuilt mechanisms for switching off desire. Unlike most other adult creatures, we are constantly dissatisfied; forever striving, seeking novelty and change, creating and wanting "more please." This greed factor is the source of our creativity but may also be the source of our destruction as a species.

It has been suggested by those who study evolution that Homo sapiens first arose—as many new species have done—from a genetic mutation. In this case it was a mutation in the chimpanzee gene, or rather in the genetic code of the creature which was the ancestor of both chimpanzees and humans. After all, the DNA of chimps and humans differs by less than 2 percent. We have far more similarities than differences.[1]

A normal baby chimp, like the babies of so many other species, is playful, adventurous and curious, forever exploring. A lover of novelty, always pushing the known boundaries, greedy for experience. Gradually, however, as the baby chimp matures, the adult instincts kick in. The love of novelty gives way to tribal routine, to limits, to territoriality and to predetermined behavior—not so, in this new mutation. Although the individuals grew to adulthood, the "switch off childhood behavior now" command never came. So here we are, playful, adventurous and curious human beings, forever exploring—first the world, then the moon, now deep space. Our love of novelty gave us our ever changing fashions, our proliferation of consumer goods, our entertainment industry. We created science, technology, the arts, the whole of our civilization, in all its myriad cultural forms, out of our inability to grow into adult chimpanzees. So our lack of an "enough" switch has made us who we are.

At the same time, it has taken—and continues to take—an ever increasing toll on the limited resources of our planetary home. This means that each one of us needs to find a way of inserting that switch into his or her life by an act of will.

The good news, however, is that there are two types of people for whom that doesn't hurt at all. One is the person whose spiritual practice is so well developed that the bliss of living each moment to the full has totally replaced the tendency to be ruled by desires. (There are few of those around, unfortunately.) The other is the elder, in this case, the elderwoman.

If the elderwoman is following the deep inner promptings of this life stage, such as the urges to simplify her life, to get rid of ballast and to spend more time in quiet reflection, it is more than likely that she will find herself having more and more delightful experiences of enoughness, just like my dinner at Daniela's.

We can encourage this process greatly by our spiritual practice. Meditative focusing on our sensory experiences not only brings us deep delight, it also helps to create that feeling of sufficiency. If you doubt this, I invite you to try an experiment. Buy a packet of the best raisins you can find. (Or if you dislike raisins, substitute something similarly sweet and chewy.) While you are watching TV or reading your library book, eat as many as you feel like eating, but leave one or two in the packet. Twenty-four hours later, do the Raisin Meditation from Chapter Nine. Notice the difference in the quality of your experience and your feeling of satisfaction.

After a few years of living with this simplicity mindset, it becomes a habit. Eventually, it is who we are. Overconsumption now looks grotesque to us. Consumerism begins to feel obscene.

The only problem is, this can set us apart from others, even from those we love, and from that set-apart place we sometimes feel lonely. But what we often do not realize is that those values of simplicity, thrift and living lightly are gradually transferring themselves in quiet and subtle ways to the world around us, especially if we just quietly live them, rather than preaching them.

A dislike of the excesses of consumerism does not mean that we should never buy anything, any more than a dislike of gluttony should put us off eating and enjoying our food. Neither should there be a need to spend time wrestling with oughts and shoulds when it comes to spending money, either on ourselves or others. For if we have truly learned to tune in to our inner wisdom and listen to what our hearts are telling us, the answer will usually be there, waiting for us. To illustrate that, let me tell you another story.

It was late November, and one of my daughters had a birthday. She was living half a world away, newly married to a man I had not yet met.

He was sitting nearby, watching, as she eagerly pounced on that morning's mail.

"And here's a card from my mother," she said, happily, slitting the envelope.

"Oh good," he said. "Does it have a check in it?"

She looked at him in surprise, the card's enclosure still in her hand. "No," she said. "It has a poem. Mom often writes me a poem for my birthday."

"Oh." He seemed disappointed. "My mom usually sends a check."

She turned, looking deeply into his eyes, and said softly, "Which would you really rather she sent you—a check or a poem?"

He thought for a while and then sighed. "A poem. But she never would."

A long time later, when I heard the story of that moment, I felt sad. I wished I could write him a poem myself. And a long time later still, after I came to know him well, I did try hard, several times, to write one for him, knowing how much he would appreciate it. But the right words would never come. I could not figure out why. It was not that my love was lacking. I had become very fond of him by then. But there is something about a poem which simply has to well up spontaneously. Trying to produce one on command, merely in order to please someone, just never seems to work—for me, anyway. Later it occurred to me that any poem I wrote him might deepen even further the sadness he felt about his own mother's apparent inability to show her love in any but material ways. And at some deep, unconscious level, perhaps I knew that. There is a certain intuitive, inexplicable rightness in things, sometimes, that I believe we must always trust.

I saw a sweater, one day, that I just knew he would love—and he did. It was expensive, and it stretched my budget. But I bought it because it felt so right. And it probably was. He wore it often.

Another time, I found a child's toy helicopter in the Salvation Army store, and I bought it for that same son-in-law, who was then learning to fly helicopters. It was all battered and scratched, and cost only fifty cents. He laughed when I gave it to him, gift-wrapped. But it became his mascot, perched on top of the desk in his study.

So I discovered, when I looked back over these various incidents, that I follow a set of guidelines for gift giving, though until then I had never thought to articulate them. I think they are as follows:

1. A gift must come directly from the heart. The only contribution the head makes is to assist with the logistics (where could I get one of those? what color matches her eyes?..., etc).
2. If a gift doesn't feel absolutely right, it isn't, no matter how logical, practical, sensible or opportune it might seem.
3. If a gift does feel absolutely right—it is.
4. The monetary value of a gift is always totally irrelevant if the love is 100 percent genuine and comes welling up like breast milk.
5. Gifts given out of habit, convention, social pressure or self-aggrandizement carry very little value or meaning. If the giver is faking the giving, the receiver will also be faking the gratitude, even if nobody lets on.

It is hard, especially at Christmas time, to go against the grain of convention. Many of us worry about the consumer ethos and the rampant spending that sweeps through at that time of year like a monsoon, often bringing devastation in its wake in the form of swollen credit cards and ruined budgets. So we search frantically for solutions. We talk about trying to find time to make our own gifts, downsizing, negotiating spending limits with family members—all sorts of techniques to bring the exchange of gifts back down to human scale and make it wonderful and meaningful again.

But perhaps we are missing something obvious and easy. And that is the fact that simplifying is always done more effectively with the heart that with the head. Tuning in is often better than figuring out. And this probably applies to a lot more things than gift-buying. It almost certainly applies to things which we want for ourselves. If we are really clear about why we want something, our hearts will usually advise us. If we can truly listen to the messages of advice from our hearts, we shall always give the right gift. And we shall always get exactly what we need for ourselves also. It will be neither too much nor too little. Like Daniela's dinner, it will be just the right amount. It will be enough.

So along with the principle of enoughness—and as a prerequisite for understanding and embracing it—is a further principle we can now add to our list. This is the principle of heart-listening. Heart-listening is to head-listening as wisdom is to knowledge.

We now have thirteen elderwoman principles. A baker's dozen.

• simplicity • deep vision • compassion • non-attachment • Earth-centeredness • comfort • connectedness • respect • creativity • delight • lightness • enoughness • heart-listening •

This last one leads me next to consideration of certain factors which are essential to good listening of any kind, and to heart-listening in particular. These are peace and quiet—and space.

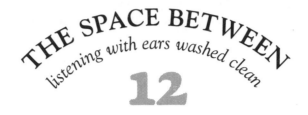

THE SPACE BETWEEN
listening with ears washed clean
12

A NEIGHBOR of mine loves to paint pictures of pebbles. Smooth, water-worn pebbles, in soft colors, with delicate tracings of quartz, each one a tiny abstract work of art.

She told me the other day that she has a new idea for presenting her work. She is going to place small pebble pictures at the center of quite large frames. The idea, she said, is that just as the eye sometimes zeroes in on one particular pebble as we walk along the beach, so will the eye travel to the center of her painting and focus more keenly there. The beauty of the pebble will thus be enhanced by the space around it.

It is the space between the notes which creates music; the space between the words is the soul of poetry; a home is the space between four walls, not the walls themselves. In the Taoist classic *Tao Te Ching*, Lao Tzu says:

> *Knead clay in order to make a vessel. Adapt the nothing*
> *therein to the purpose in hand and you will have the use of*
> *the vessel. Cut out doors and windows in order to make a*
> *room. Adapt the nothing therein to the purpose in hand*
> *and you will have the use of the room.*

Thus what we gain is Something, yet it is by virtue of Nothing that this can be put to use.[1]

In Eastern ways of thinking, the Nothing has as much substance and validity as the Something which replaces it. Any Something we create is going to displace some of that important Nothing, and therefore we have to choose carefully our placement of things.

In all our human communication, the meanings of our spoken messages are conveyed not merely by the words but also in a dozen other subtle ways. Body language, voice tone and inflection, facial expressions, etc., all use the spaces between and around the words themselves to convey meaning. We often refer to "reading between the lines," in other words, reading the deeper meaning between the words. But if the lines are too thickly placed upon the page and there is no space between them, the result is mental indigestion.

It might seem strange to talk about the Nothing which the Something replaces as though it were an entity rather than merely the absence of an entity. An element of Eastern philosophy which often puzzles Westerners is the whole notion of what Buddhists call the Void. To us, empty space is just that—empty space. In our culture, it is something to fill up. If we ever pause to wonder why a newly painted blank wall so quickly becomes covered in graffiti, it may occur to us that our young folk are simply reflecting our whole culture's greedy tendency to use up anything it sees as blank space. A niche, a marketing opportunity, an unfilled desire, all these are eagerly sought after by those bent on filling them. The Nothing, in our culture, is scarcely valued at all. There is Muzak in the elevator, TV in the departure lounge, commercials between programs, pop-ups on web sites and ads on buses and taxicabs. At the movies, these days we rarely sit looking at the elegant fold of a vast, red velvet curtain in a proscenium arch, noticing the other people as they come in, and quietly anticipating the pleasures to come. We have to watch advertisements for nearby pizza restaurants instead. There was a time, not so many years ago, when airlines showed long-haul passengers a couple of movies and then the screen went dark and passengers slept—or tried to. Not now. The programs are more often than not continuous, and people trying to sleep have to find their own ways of blotting out the flickering light of the video screen. We walk along the street talking on our cell phones or listening to music on our Walkmen. Even out on the trails, deep in the woods, I see people with headphones clamped fast to their ears. More and more, year by year, we are squeezing out that all important space between. We are greedy for the Something, but we have forgotten how to honor the Nothing out of which it is created. So the Something is slowly choking us to death. For if Something and Nothing are not in balance—equally honored—then our world is out of kilter. And when our world is out of kilter we get sick.

Whether we get sick physically or mentally, emotionally or spiritually is immaterial. They are all interconnected anyway.

One of the marks of an elderwoman is that she feels the discomfort of this, at some level. She feels, in her own psyche, that squeezing pressure, that feeling of threat to her own vital space between. Whether or not she has understood or articulated it, matters not. The important thing is that she has picked up the feeling that there is something wrong and is casting about for ways to redress the balance. She may find herself turning off the TV because she can no longer bear the bombardment of noise and information, the banality, the relentless barrage of commercialism and violence in all its forms. She may find that she no longer enjoys a night at the movies because it is too loud, too violent, too uncomfortable. She may find herself increasingly reluctant to visit the shopping mall because of the feeling of being assailed by noise and chaos and the pressure to consume. She may have walked out of a store, or even a restaurant, because the music was so loud that she could no longer think clearly. Where the vast array of goods in the supermarket might once have excited her, these days she may be starting to find it more sickening and confusing than it is exciting.

She might sigh and blame herself. "Oh it must be just that I am getting old," she'll say.

Yes, she is right. It *is* because she is getting old. But let's examine the feeling which goes with that thought. An old woman's feeling could be expressed as "I am getting old. That means I am getting towards the end of my life. I am finding it harder and harder to adjust to society. Ho-hum, that's the way it goes—nothing I can do about it." The elderwoman's feeling, on the other hand, expresses itself as "I am getting old. That means I'm at the stage of my life where I can see a lot of the ways in which our society has gone wrong. I need to bear witness to this feeling, in whatever way I can, even if only to acknowledge it to myself. Hey-ho, that's my task now."

That pretty well sums up the main difference between an old woman and an elderwoman. The former still believes that she has no power and therefore no alternative but to adjust herself to her society. The elderwoman, by contrast, is empowered. Not by the granting of that power to her by anyone else, but simply by the power which flows from her own confidence in being who she is. From her deep knowing that she, as an elder, now has the wisdom to do her share of the guiding of her society, the experience to know what needs changing and the right to let her voice be heard.

Men seem to have less difficulty with that. Centuries of patriarchy have, I believe, built into them a much greater sense of personal empowerment. And despite the fact that many older men find themselves sidelined by the corporate world and many of them experience similar dissatisfactions with the way things are, reluctance to speak out has never been a such a problem for them as it has for many women. This, in case any reader is wondering, is one of the reasons why this book is about the elderwoman, not elders in general. (Another reason being, of course, that I believe there are significant differences between the male and female psyche, and it is the female psyche which interests me more.)

This tendency to fill up all the available spaces makes it more and more difficult for us to tune in to the things we need to hear and understand in order to bring our world back into balance. It is a vicious circle. The more out of balance the world is—the more Somethings that are crammed in to squeeze out the Nothing—the more noise and chaos there is—then the less ability we have to tune into that last remaining bit of Nothing, and the harder it is to listen for answers. For answers come out of the quiet spaces—out of the Nothing, in other words. Just as you cannot hear a cricket chirp in the middle of a busy intersection, you cannot easily listen for inner wisdom when there is so much chaos swirling around you. When there is a lot of static, you lose the ability to hear the subtler levels of communication from others also. You may hear their shouted words; may pick up the feelings from seeing their body language, but with so much to filter out, you are less able to tune right into them and hear the subtle layers of their messages. You may intuit their feeling tone, particularly if they are angry, unhappy or depressed, but instead of resonating with it and perhaps homing in on what really might be going on with them, it simply registers in you as a general feeling of discomfort. It is only against a peaceful background that we can truly listen to each other. When the TV is blaring, or people are hurrying between appointments, trying to juggle too many activities or living in messy, cluttered spaces, the background against which we are living is not conducive to really good communication. Like a hasty, half-digested meal, such interactions with others will feel neither good nor satisfying.

If we cannot even hear, against all that static, the subtleties of communication from other living beings, how much less able are we to tune into any other possible energies which may surround us. Whether we call them spirits, angels, discarnate entities, telepathic communications or whatever, it seems clear that for some people it is possible to pursue communications which lie outside the generally accepted wavebands of science and our five senses. This should not be surprising. Most of us have seen evidence that other animals are able to do this, so why not us? Anyone who has shared a house with a dog will know that you only have to think "Oh it is sunny now, I think I'll go for a walk" and a sleeping dog will wake up and leap to its feet with expectant barks of joy, even though you have neither spoken the thought aloud nor moved a muscle. Even though we can neither comprehend nor explain these non-material energies and phenomena, we need to recognize and honor them, and to leave space between our thoughts and actions so that they can come in.

It is necessary to look at our physical surroundings also. As I remarked in Chapter 3, when my desk is cluttered, my mind is cluttered. Karen Kingston, who has authored several popular books on feng-shui, points out that many people miss the whole point and go for a quick-fix. Feng-shui, the ancient Oriental art of placement, which, above all other disciplines, pays great heed to the space between, is not just a technique for improving your prosperity or health, but a philosophy of life which honors the need to balance Something with Nothing. By ignoring these basic ideas and simply hanging up wind-chimes, we often unwittingly create more problems than we solve. As Kingston reminds us, if you hang a mirror in a corner of your bedroom but the corner is full of clutter, then all you will do is double the clutter—and with it, the chaos in your life![2]

Possibly one of the reasons feng shui has now become so popular in the West, is that we are finally realizing how little consideration our culture has given to the art of balance and the juxtaposition of objects with space. Even if many people do not fully understand the cure for this, at least they are groping intuitively towards it.

Just as with the static that drowns out sound, if we fill our lives with too much stuff, we no longer have the ability to see anything properly. I can remember, as a child, being taken to the Natural History Museum in London, and because of the wartime air raids a lot of things had been hastily taken out of their displays and were all crammed in, higgledy-piggledy, in basement rooms. I stared uncomprehendingly at this jumble of objects. Nothing made sense. It was all too much to take in, and very unsatisfying.

That helps me to realize that by cluttering our houses with consumer goods, we lose the space that gives our most special things the frame they need in order to be properly seen and appreciated.

By cramming sound and chatter and activity into every available crevice in our lives, many of us unintentionally fill up all that all-important space between, which gives our activities their deepest meaning. I heard someone remark recently that most people are deeply afraid of silence. And yet silence is the necessary frame for sound. Music that was not surrounded by silence would no longer be music, but would become a relentless assault of noise upon our ears.

Not only are we not able fully to hear music or each other against the Something-filled background, but we are not able to listen clearly to ourselves either. In order to develop our elderwoman capacities to the full, and be able to hear the soft voice of our own intuition so that we may channel wisdom into the world, periods of calm and silence are essential. It is of increasing importance to the elderwoman, as she ages, to reclaim that precious space.

Not only do we need more silence as we get older but many of us enjoy it more. At times, nowadays, I find myself craving it.

My grandmother appeared to have enjoyed it too, though maybe not in a conscious way. Like many other things, it would have been a taken-for-granted part of her life. There was less traffic then. The world was a quieter place. She had no TV, video or Internet. For many years she had no telephone. She listened to the radio sometimes, and she sang songs to herself and hummed as she worked. But often, in the evenings, she would sit quietly sewing, while my grandfather read his library book, and the only sound in the room was the ticking of the big wooden clock on the mantelpiece.

There is something about the ticking of an old-fashioned clock which seems to deepen the silence around it, in the same way that a gong can deepen meditation and the sanctus bell deepens prayer. Deep silence, when you really learn to listen to it, is one of the most wonderful, soothing and joyous things there is. First, however, we have to let go of our noisy habits and learn to hear properly again.

Brother David Steindl-Rast, in his book of essays entitled *A Listening Heart*, speaks of visiting a remote mission school in Australia's Northern Territory run by the Sisters of St Joseph. He notes how the sisters protected the inner silence of the children entrusted to their care. They taught the children outside, rather than in the schoolroom, teaching them through their mothers, in respect for the traditional culture of those desert people. They spoke softly, using images in preference to words. Nonetheless, says Brother David,

> *School must have seemed like an avalanche of words to these*
> *children. At recess time between classes, they utterly surprised*
> *me. I was used to pupils bursting out into the schoolyard,*
> *yelling and hollering. These children… walked out into the*
> *surrounding bush in complete silence, as if to wash their ears*
> *clean from too much talk.*[3]

I like that notion of washing our ears clean. For with "clean" ears, we can really begin to hear silence and to pay full attention to the subtle sounds which may otherwise have passed unnoticed. Then sounds will come into relief against the quiet, like pictures freshly framed: birdsong; the cricket's chirp; that evening creaking that houses do, as they contract after a day in the sun.

In the peacefulness of a country night, we hear the distant hoot of an owl or the fox's wheezy bark and our senses expand, reaching out into the darkness, alert, alive. But when our ears are assailed by the cacophony of daytime in the city—the roar of traffic, the relentless dribble of Muzak, and the noises of all our machines, from dishwashers and vacuum cleaners to trucks and chainsaws, not to mention a thousand chattering human voices, both live and electronic—it is hard not to shut down.

In shut-down mode, with senses dulled, we sleepwalk, out of touch with the world around us. Ironically, we may feel safer, because that very dulling removes our inner life from our awareness also. If people fear silence it is usually because in silence they can no longer avoid confronting the thoughts and memories they have been suppressing, or feeling the feelings they may have long denied. Silence creates inner space, and some of what rushes in to fill that space may be unwelcome. There is no way around this. The only way is through it.

Most people, when they first begin a meditation practice, find that personal issues soon start rising to the surface. However, if we are able simply to sit in pure awareness of feeling and emotion, without engaging the chattering mind—like hearing the music but ignoring the lyrics—then eventually, we find ourselves borne on the current of meditation out of the realm of either thought or feeling, into a deep place of true peace and silence.

It is in silence that the work of integration takes place. Information which we have taken in cannot become part of us until we have had time and space to integrate it, just as food cannot nourish us until it has had a chance to be peacefully digested. Insights often cannot be gained until we sit quietly and look back on our lived experience. Neither can the necessary perspective be achieved. This becomes increasingly important as we get older and more naturally reflective. In order for our accumulated wisdom to be of benefit to others, it needs a quiet and beautiful space in which to be distilled, and one of the tasks of the elderwoman is to create that space in whatever way best expresses her true, individual nature. In this way, as we saw in Chapter 8, her home, the arrangement of her possessions and her very life combine to become her personal, unique work of art.

The older I get, and the more I appreciate silence, the better I understand that thing which always puzzled me as a child: why my grandmother loved to sit so quietly in that chair. I know, now, what she was doing. She was simply enjoying the space between, listening with ears washed clean.

When we wash our ears clean and attune once more to the sweet sound of silence, that is when we might finally begin to hear the harmonics of the Universe, the mystical descant of angel voices which silence brings to all who truly listen. It is certainly worth a try.

So in order to follow a number of the elderwoman principles, particularly deep vision, heart-listening, comfort and delight, peace and quiet is now more important to us than ever before. In fact, it is essential. So I shall add it to our list as a principle in its own right.

• simplicity • deep vision • compassion • non-attachment •
• Earth-centeredness • comfort • connectedness • respect • creativity •
• delight • lightness • enoughness • heart-listening • peace and quiet •

TRAVELING LIGHT
tips for the conscious traveler
13

AFTER TWELVE months of working, we earn a vacation. So right now, after twelve chapters, and before we leave the air element, seems an appropriate moment to consider how the elderwoman might approach the whole question of travel. Many of us find travel exciting and hope to continue as long as we can. But there is another aspect to that excitement.

I remember my first ever trip to New York City. It was late in the evening when I had my first glimpse of the skyscrapers of Manhattan. The DC10 dropped below the clouds, and suddenly there we were, surrounded by a fairyland of spangled lights; a Christmas tree world stretching to infinity. It felt almost unreal.

Later, from my way-up-there hotel room I looked down into the sleepless streets, felt the buzz, felt the energy of the city that throbs and hums its way around the clock, never sleeping, never resting. New York pulses with a vitality which, when you first sense it, is almost shocking in its rawness. Remembering that experience, and how I dealt with it, has set me thinking about what sorts of techniques I have used over the years to keep my balance and maintain, in all manner of settings, the simple, quiet, reflective style of life I find so satisfying.

I think there are two ways to go, especially in a place which has such a different energy from the places you are used to. Either you ride it, surf on the back of the excitement, let it carry you, and run the risk of crashing, or you duck quietly under it, take it in small doses, pace yourself carefully, rest a lot.

To ride it is to take a huge risk, for in a way it is like a drug. Our bodies and our psyches can only take so much of that kind of stress without rebounding into the automatic protective shutdown of the organism, which manifests as exhaustion, illness, depression or an unreal dream state. On that first visit to New York, being much younger then, I rode the wave, and paid for it with a spaciness that split me off from awareness of my body. That, and other experiences, have taught me that the better option—especially when we are older and less resilient—is to stay very aware of the impact of a new place, and open to it gradually, gently.

What I believe we should never do is try to fight that unfamiliar energy or ignore it, since that causes us to contract. Contraction creates tension in our bodies, discomfort in our minds and starvation for our souls, which yearn to interact, to live fully and juicily every day, through the minds and bodies which give them form.

I believe that when travelers in foreign lands become ill, often the cause may not be in the strange food, the local water and the unfamiliar bacteria, but rather in the failure to acknowledge the differential energy of place and adjust to it slowly and carefully, without shutting down or spacing out.

If we are careful at the beginning, accustoming ourselves gradually to the newness, while staying fully aware, alive and open to the world around us, then travel takes on a different dimension.

I have found that for me, the best trick is to create a safe, quiet haven, from which to come and go. A hotel room can be perfect for this. To make it so, we need to keep the room peaceful, and to do whatever practice we normally use to quiet and center ourselves. There are many little things which help this process. a herbal pillow from home; a meditation shawl; a familiar brand of bottled water; our journals; keeping a food stash, so we are not forced out to the cafe or restaurant when we are weary.

Each time we return to that haven and center ourselves and our energy, we can reflect on the feelings which have been stirred within us by our forays, assimilate our experiences, and overcome all the little shocks of difference and unfamiliarity.

The more aware we are of our inner moment-by-moment responses to the new experiences, the better we can pace ourselves, and therefore the greater our enjoyment of those new experiences will be. As soon as we feel ourselves spacing out or contracting, that is a sign to head back to our haven and regroup.

Traveling this way, we allow ourselves really to see and hear and feel and be touched by the places we visit and the people we meet, rather than staring at them as we would a video. They become three-dimensional. They become our teachers. As we let these new teachings in, we expand, change and grow as a result. That, surely, is what travel is really about. Otherwise we may as well have saved our money, stayed home, watched films about other places and read travel books.

So let us look a bit more closely at what happens to us when we travel. Those of us who like to live with dogs and cats know the difficulties they have with change and unfamiliarity. Yet we tend to think of ourselves as being above such difficulties. After all, traveling, especially going on vacation, is one of the things most of us look forward to with great pleasure.

There is a well-known scale in psychology known as the Holmes and Rahe Stress Scale, which lists stressful occurrences in the average human life according to their relative severity and the comparative degree of toll they take on the human organism. In number one place—worth one hundred points on the scale—is the death of one's most significant other. Divorce scores seventy-three. A jail term is worth sixty-three and getting fired from work rates forty-seven. Obviously, many of the stressors on the list are painful, sad and uncomfortable things, but not all. Marriage, for example, which for most brides and grooms is a particularly happy occasion, still causes wear and tear on their stress-coping mechanisms and carries a stress score of fifty. Vacations, which we think of as antidotes to stress ("ah, what you really need is a break—take a vacation") actually score thirteen on the scale, one point ahead of Christmas, another ostensibly happy time, which is, according to the Holmes and Rahe Scale, slightly more stressful than being charged with a minor violation of the law![1]

Most creatures are to some extent territorial, even those whose territory spans a large area or who travel long distances between one part of their territory and another. When the swallows reappear each spring at the top of the hill, near my house, I can safely predict that they will sit on exactly the same wires as they habitually sat on every day of the previous summer and nest in exactly the same places. I believe that we, too, have territorial tendencies and become stressed whenever we are on unfamiliar ground, just as our dogs and cats do.

We should not think of stress per se as being a negative thing, for, in fact, it is a neutral process. It can have positive and negative connotations, depending on the situation. It is stress on the poles and guy ropes which keep a tent in place, for example. Without stress, it would simply be a messy pile of fabric lying on the grass. In order for us to stand upright, some of our muscle fibers have to contract and shorten while others have to relax and lengthen. Without some stress on the fibers in a piece of elastic, pants would come tumbling down around ankles worldwide. Stress and tension are natural and essential processes. They are an integral part of life.

So what we need to look at is not stress as such but the effects of various outside factors, like the ones on the Holmes and Rahe Scale, upon our bodies and minds. These are known as stressors. So in terms of travel, unfamiliarity is in itself a stressor. Whether it frighten or excites us, intrigues or delights us is immaterial. Regardless of our emotional response, we are still being in some way stirred up.

Our bodies are beautifully constructed to handle being stirred up by outside stressors, just as an automobile has shock absorbers to lessen the wear and tear on the vehicle and avoid its passengers being shaken to bits. There is a sequence of bodily events which results from even the slightest disturbance to physical equilibrium, and we call this the stress response. At its base is the well-known "fight or flight" mechanism, an automatic response of most creatures, including ourselves. Different creatures favor different aspects of this response. Step on the tail of a rattlesnake and you'll encounter a fight response you will never forget. A bird, a mouse or an antelope will never stay around long enough to fight. Other creatures, rather than either fight or flight, have specialized in "freeze" (stay so still the enemy will think you are part of the landscape and overlook you). All the methods work—most of the time—which is why they are still with us. And all of them *are* still with us. I know a woman who longed for years to go to India. When she finally did, the impact was so intense that she cut short her trip and headed home. She took flight—literally! But for those who do not take that literal option, there is a spaciness which happens, a flight out of the body. Other people, faced with the stress of unfamiliar territory, get unusually grumpy and reactive. When my partner and I backpacked across the world for eight months, we had a minor disagreement almost every day we were on the road. There are some tourists who continually pick fights with waiters, hotel clerks, flight attendants and the like. They, too, are probably exhibiting the fight response as a way of relieving their particular travel stress. And for those who render themselves immobile, either by a new and overwhelming timidity that makes them suddenly scared to venture out of the hotel, or simply by becoming ill, freezing appears to be the method of choice.

All these methods serve, as nature intended they should, to reduce stress and bring the body back into equilibrium. Understanding that process—what it is and why it happens—can not only help us to understand the typical responses we have to unfamiliar places and other travel experiences but can also assist us in finding ways around the problem and thereby making our travel more meaningful.

We should not underestimate the extra energy it takes to be in a new place. Have you vacationed in a rented cabin? Remember how much more effort it took you to cook a meal when you had to search for the right pan, locate a sharp knife, fiddle with unfamiliar knobs? Think about how weary you felt after the first day of a new job. Or how overwhelmed you were by all the things you had to learn on your first driving lesson. Our minds are so efficient at storing frequently used information and keeping it handy for us, that we can do a million things without even thinking about them. When did you last think consciously about changing gears or locating your toothpaste?

In unfamiliar places, most of the advantage of that automatic patterning is lost and we need to think about almost everything we do. Lost, too, are many of the codes that simplify our lives in familiar places, and the stranger the places are, the fewer of those codes will survive. In your home town, you know exactly where and how to mail a letter. Drive to another city. You will quickly find the mailbox because if this is the U.S.A., your eye is trained to recognize that familiar blue shape and eagle motif. Fly to London, and suddenly the mailboxes are a different shape— and they are all red. Fly to Athens and they turn yellow.

It all takes energy. So we get extra weary while we are traveling. While young people have energy to spare, we older ones have to husband ours a little more carefully, and we need to plan our days with this in mind.

Sounds reasonable, doesn't it?

Wait—there is another, subtle elderwoman difference here. The trouble with this approach (the "you kids go off and party—we old folks need to get an early night, ha ha" approach) is that it is focused on what we cannot do rather than what we can and on who we no longer are rather than what we have newly become. It is focused on loss rather than gain, i.e. on the loss of strength and stamina rather than the gaining of depth, understanding, compassion, wisdom and joy.

For the elderwoman, travel to new and different places is an opportunity to feast at new tables. As she gets older, even though she may remain very physically fit, she gradually slows down. And as she slows down, she sees more—and differently. More deeply. By the very slowness with which she drinks in the scene, by the quiet, reflective way she watches, notes detail, listens for resonances between what her eyes are taking in and what her heart is feeling, her soul is being fed, in every moment. She is learning, growing, assimilating, linking what she sees to what she already knows, making connections. She sees the universal in the particular and the particular in the universal. She watches in fascination, like a child, yet the wisdom of her years enhances her understanding of all that she sees.

I remember sitting by an open window in the Nepalese capital of Katmandu, resting after my exploration of the old city, weary from all the color and bustle and activity of the street, the kaleidoscope of sounds and smells. So weary, in fact, that I decided to spend the remainder of the afternoon in, reading a book and resting. Before me, was a panorama of rooftops. As I sat gazing at this with half-closed eyes, I noticed that on one nearby rooftop, a mother was singing to her baby. Near her, a little girl played. Another scene caught my eye. A woman, on a different rooftop, was cooking a meal. Gradually, as I sat there watching, I realized that almost every rooftop was being used for some activity or another. There were whole lives being lived up there. The more I watched, the more I saw. There were old people, young people, children sleeping, working, playing, talking. Stories everywhere. Human life in microcosm.

Another time, snorkeling over a coral reef, I discovered that if, instead of swimming about, I floated motionless in one position, gazing at the display of sea life below me, more and more fascinating details of it appeared.

It does not matter where we are. Any scene, if we gaze at it long enough, will reveal deeper and deeper layers of information. The inquiring mind can function either as a telescope, straining to see farther and farther out into the cosmos, or as a microscope, peering ever more deeply within. When we are young, we travel with telescope mind, gathering up wide swathes of information as we go, sweeping the heavens for knowledge. As elderwomen, we travel now with microscope mind, knowing that the more we look at something, the more we shall see and the wiser we shall become.

So to travel in a light and simple way is not only to travel with minimal luggage (because we have learned to carry around only what is really necessary and because we dress for comfort) but also to dip lightly into the newness, to sip it and savor it like never before.

It is also to travel consciously, to be aware of our impact on the places and people we visit. Much modern tourism, unfortunately, causes pollution, environmental damage, water shortage and social disruption; so we should be mindful of this before we book tickets. During World War II, there was a poster which asked "Is your journey really necessary?" Maybe we should put that up again. I sometimes feel guilty about all the oil my adventures have used up, over the years. But I do treasure those memories.

When I look back, the times I most enjoy remembering are not so much those where I simply gazed in awe at beautiful scenery or gasped in amazement at feats of architecture. They are those where I interacted, either with the landscape itself, or with people.

Like the day we took the ferry from Greece to Turkey. I can see it now, the little boat from Rhodes, flying its red Turkish crescent and star, nudging into the colorful floating world of Marmaris harbor.

There were so many boats. So many unusual shapes, sizes and designs jostling for attention that it was hard to concentrate on the serious business of coming ashore. It was, after all, an international arrival, complete with passports—passports which we did (thank goodness) get back out of that frighteningly informal-looking cardboard box which someone brought aboard in Rhodes and placed on an old wooden chair in the middle of the deck.

Beyond the harbor, the town itself beckoned, with its jumble of old and new, modern hotels and graceful minarets. In the center, like a pulsing heart, were the narrow, crowded, canvas-shaded streets that make up the traditional Turkish bazaar. Its air smelled of spices. Its stalls bulged with delights: burnished copper jugs, colorful tapestries, tubs of saffron, hookahs of brass and colored glass, ornaments and bells, cushions and toys.

At the bakery, I was delighted to find simits—delicious crusty circlets of bread coated with sesame seeds—and I remember slipping one on my wrist like a bangle, and munching another as we walked in search of interesting accommodation.

It was not hard to find. Soon we were installed in our simple, inexpensive rooftop quarters on top of someone's house. A little building on the roof housed a bed and an electric light. Outside, under a reed awning, was a table and chairs. A tiny lean-to kitchen and bathroom completed the picture. On all sides, the view was magnificent. I dubbed it "The Penthouse."

That night it rained. And rained and rained and rained.

Early next morning, waking to the muezzin's call, we looked out over a clear, washed world. Everything in sight was sodden. The heavy canvas roofs of the bazaar were drenched and drooping, and everywhere the stall holders were surveying the damage, tipping water out of the dripping pockets of canvas, sweeping puddles.

There were no visitors around yet. Only us. We sloshed through the wet street, smiling good morning, and everyone smiled back. They pointed at the water, they laughed and made wry faces. We laughed and made wry faces back. There was a camaraderie in the air, as they helped each other clean up, and I suddenly felt part of a different world—a backstage world, where the props got all wet in the night and everyone laughs together at calamity.

At the bakery, there were fresh simits on the counter. The baker smiled and beckoned us through to the back of his shop. He motioned towards chairs. We sat, and he brought us tiny fragrant cups of apple tea, and one for himself. We knew no Turkish except a basic greeting and he knew no English except hello, but it did not matter. We sat in companionable silence, drinking tea.

As we were leaving, he put a finger to his lips. Grinning, he pointed silently to the huge brick oven, empty now and cooling off from last night's baking. We peered in. Just inside, curled up fast asleep, lay his young, flour-dusted apprentice. We all laughed together, in shared, wordless amusement.

Looking back, later, I tried to figure out what it was about Marmaris that made the delight factor so strong. Eventually it dawned on me that the whole experience, from start to finish had been human-sized.

From the cardboard box of passports, through the displays of touchable, feelable items in the bazaar, the simplicity of our accommodation, and the camaraderie of that wet morning, to the hospitality of the baker and the funny, touching sight of the sleeping apprentice, everything was human-sized, human-shaped—and interactive. No machines, no computer screens, no plate glass windows, shrink-wrap packaging, hotel lobbies or bus windows separated us from the life around us. We were in it and of it.

I am not a total Luddite. I love computers, videos and my power drill. I thrill at the elegance of human-made marvels like the Golden Gate Bridge. An hour spent surfing the Internet can dazzle my mind with information. But in another hour, most of that is gone again. The things that stay with me are always the simple, human-sized, interactive things. They are the memories that linger on, fragrant as the smell of cinnamon, crunchy as a simit, funny as an oven with a sleeping boy curled up inside.

These are elderwoman memories, the joys of which become richer in the retelling. It is these we travel to find, bring home and think about, with deepening delight, in the long winter evenings. And it is these which will continue to delight and nourish us when we can no longer physically leave home and our only travel takes place within.

This is part of the harvest.

fire

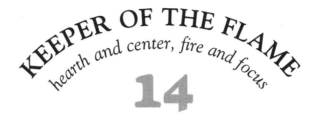

KEEPER OF THE FLAME
hearth and center, fire and focus
14

AS WE TURN, now, to the fire element, I want to talk first about Hestia.

I often find myself thinking of her, these days. The goddess Hestia was, as you probably know, the Greek goddess of the hearth, worshiped in every household and temple. She was addressed thus:

> *Hestia, in the high dwellings of all, both deathless gods and*
> *men who walk on earth, you have gained an everlasting*
> *abode and highest honor: glorious is your portion and your*
> *right. For without you mortals hold no banquet — where*
> *one does not duly pour sweet wine in offering to Hestia*
> *both first and last.*[1]

While the other gods romped around the world, getting their noses into everything, Hestia remained quietly at home, so we hear no stories of her in mythology. Neither were any images of her produced. The Romans called her Vesta, and her priestesses—who attended the eternal flame that burned day and night in her honor—the Vestal Virgins.

As I move further into elderhood, Hestia has become important. While I still enjoy travel and adventure, I find myself growing increasingly appreciative of the gentle quietude and comfort to be found close to my hearth and home. And as I rest into that, it reveals to me more and more of its sacred nature.

Like my grandmother, I have no central heating in my living room; just this wonderful wood-burning stove, through whose glass front I can watch the flames lick and curl around the logs. In the evenings, when all else is still, those dancing flames are the focal point of the whole room as their warmth reaches out to embrace us.

"Focus," the Latin word for fireplace, for hearth, for the central place around which our lives revolve. The semantics are interesting. And the words "heart" and "hearth" sound so similar, even though their etymological origins differ.

We have a deep human need for a warm center, whether it be our own open hearts, the central hearth in our dwelling place, or the central focal point in cities, towns and villages. The heart/hearth is where the goddess dwells. Her sacred breath is what turns a humble task into a meditation, a conversation into a dance of souls, a house into a home, and a group of people into a community.

A friend who recently relocated to one of those "new towns" on the outer edge of a city sprawl wrote to me in puzzlement, "I keep looking for the 'heart' of this place, the town square or gathering place, and I haven't found it."

I know how she feels. I lived in a place like that myself, once. Like her, I went looking for the heart. Eventually the awful truth dawned. There wasn't one. As Gertrude Stein once said, "I went there, but there wasn't any 'there' there."

In many towns, the center has been replaced by the shopping mall. In the centrally heated home, the hearth has largely been replaced by the television set as the focal point of the room. And within our own beings, the heart center can so easily be overshadowed by the solar plexus—the power center—where we experience our own clutching desire for control and for material possessions. It is no mere coincidence that these things—power, the TV commercials and the shopping mall—are connected.

It often seems as though money has replaced the Great Spirit. And yet I believe that within the hearts of people, a flame still burns, guarded night and day by Hestia's priestesses. Polls and sociological surveys designed to measure the true extent of materialistic values in ordinary people's lives consistently discover that such values are only skin deep. At heart, we want to interact, to gather around the fire and tell our stories, to dance together in the square, to feast, and pour the "sweet wine."

This becomes particularly apparent at Christmas time. You do not need a team of sociologists, with clipboards, to find out how people feel about the commercial takeover of this once-simple communal celebration. Anyone you ask will tell you. Almost anyone over the age of fifty will reminisce, with a nostalgic sigh, about how much nicer Christmas used to be, "in the old days," when the emphasis was more on the celebration of Christ's birth, and less on getting and having. That birth brought a new light to the world, metaphorically speaking, just as the solstice—the turning point of midwinter—brings the promise that light will return, now that the longest night is past. So the fusion of these two traditions, one two thousand years old and the other many times older, has created for us northern hemisphere dwellers a rich opportunity for celebration. Yet even though the candles get brighter and the street decorations more elaborate, many people feel that Christmas is somehow spoiled, nowadays. By contrast, I never hear anyone say that about Thanksgiving, a ritual which has for the most part escaped commercialization and managed to retain its heart values.

I believe, too, that the arts of a society give very clear clues to what that society's deepest values really are. Over and over again, in our movies, it is still the heart values which win out, despite the endless scenes of brutality and shootings and car chases. We understood, without explanation, the importance of "The Force." Watching *Field of Dreams* we all knew, didn't we, that had we been there, we, too, would have seen the ghostly players on the field? Naturally we would. How many of us aligned ourselves with the bad guys who stared in puzzlement at the empty field and saw only real estate? Not one, I bet, including the realtors in the audience.

So despite the fact that our world is getting despoiled at a terrifying rate, that global warming is now a frightening reality and the rainforests continue to be chopped down, that people, nature and the Earth's resources continue to be exploited in the name of profit and a few rich people get richer while more and more millions live in poverty, I really do not believe this is because there are "bad" people and "good" people. I think it is because many people in powerful places have become so busy and distracted that they spend very little time at their own hearths. By which I mean that they have left no quiet spaces in which to meditate and think deeply. They have deprived themselves of the opportunity to reflect, to ponder, to get in touch with the full implications of their actions on the world and whether or not these are in tune with their own heart values. Or they have allowed their minds to be swayed by the philosophies or promises of others, swallowing ideas whole without feeling into the rightness of those ideas at soul level.

Then there are countless others, possibly the majority, who have gotten themselves trapped by their own needs, wants and desires into working for the "system" even when their hearts are not in tune with the end results that system creates. If I were a logger whose heart ached at the felling of a tree but for whom the job with the woodchip company was the only way I could earn enough to feed my kids, would I still cut the tree? Chances are, I would close down that tender part of myself, cover the wound with reassurance, change my stated beliefs, because not to do so would be to live with an inner dissonance so painful that it would make me ill.

Many of us who weep and shout the loudest about the crisis in our planet's ecosystem, or about human injustice, are people who have not had to make such difficult choices, people who have not had to give up a great deal in order to be green. And we know that if all the world were to be green, and resources were to be fairly shared, quite a lot of people would have to give up heaps. So we should hesitate before we condemn others for the state of the world. At the very least we should be certain, before we pass judgment on anyone else, that we ourselves are beyond reproach. If I feel outraged because a certain multinational company has blatantly discouraged Indian women from breast-feeding their children in order to increase the sales of its formula feed and make millions, there is little I can say about it while I am still buying that company's coffee or chocolate because they are the cheapest ones in the supermarket, or still investing my money in such a way that I, too, profit from such sales, however indirectly. If I am not prepared to pay more for fair-traded, shade-grown coffee, or for chocolate made from fair-traded cocoa beans—or go without—and if I do not have the energy to trace all the uses to which my savings might be put or the willingness to drop a percentage point in interest in order to ensure a more ethical use of my money, then I should be careful before I cast the first stone.

All I can do, in that case, is simply to share my predicament honestly with others. I can be open about my falling short of my own ideal. I can own my fallibility, my ambivalence, my shame and my desire to try harder. When it comes to being greener, this is the category into which most of us fall.

Perhaps one of the most difficult parts of the elderwoman's role is her growing inner need to check and measure everything in her life against those deepest heart values. Any component of our daily lives, any item we buy, any statement we make is likely to trigger in us the questions that so many other people do not appear to stop and ask themselves. Is this good for me? Is this good for my loved ones, for the world's children and their children's children's children? Is this item/action/statement causing any hurt or injustice to anyone or any creature, anywhere? Does this really feel, deep down, like an OK thing to do/buy/say?

But once Hestia, the goddess of the hearth, begins to make her presence felt in our lives and we start living more and more from the heart, it becomes increasingly difficult *not* to ask the questions. This can sometimes feel like a lonely road, especially when one is surrounded by others for whom the questions rarely arise and for whom the expediency of the moment—or the need to join in with the latest fad or fashion—appears the only important thing. The elderwoman sitting by her hearth, in deep contemplation of the world she has lived in so long and come to know and love so well, cannot help but take a longer view. Her longer view may lead to the issuing of warnings and cautions to those who cannot see further back than twenty years or further ahead than the end of the week and are ignorant of the dangers lurking behind their decisions.

In older, more traditional tribal cultures, this thoughtful conservatism of the elders was often a highly valued thing, a necessary protection against repeating mistakes of the past. It is the accumulated wisdom of the elders, rather than the memory of one single individual, which takes account of the hundred-year flood and picks a building site a little higher up the hillside.

Rabbi Schachter-Shalomi, who founded the Spiritual Eldering Institute in Philadelphia, conjures up an interesting image of how it feels to come into the presence of someone in whom the "elder" aspect is fully developed. He says it is like taking an elevator to the top floor of a skyscraper where there is a revolving restaurant.

Sipping a cup of tea as the restaurant makes an unhurried revolution every hour, we contemplate the landscape for miles in each direction because of our enlarged perspective. When we return to the hustle and bustle or life below, we carry this wider vision into our daily transactions.[2]

This image of soaring above the Earth in order to see a far distance brings to mind something a friend showed me recently. It was a wonderful collection of photographs taken from Space, accompanied by the words of numerous astronauts, both U.S. and Russian. It is clear, from reading their accounts of their experiences in Space and the profound change it wrought in their way of seeing the world, that the opportunity to see Earth from that incredible distance was for all of them a transformative experience.

Hestia's hearth, on the other hand, is an archetypally feminine image. In Hestia's tradition, the hearth pit was the place of entry to the underworld, where the spirits of the ancestors dwelled. So it was—as so many feminine spiritual images are—an image of going deeper and deeper down to find wisdom, rather than higher and higher up. This echoes the ancient Sumerian story of Innana, the queen who journeyed to the underworld to find her shadow sister and was first destroyed and then transformed by the process. My many years of clinical practice as a therapist, together with my own personal experiences, have left me in no doubt that as women, we typically discover our true selves by going in and down. Down, into the depths of ourselves, often down into depression, and down, sometimes, into the sheer ordinariness of everyday life. Many of us who have been housewives and mothers can probably remember the time when our only choice seemed to be to find a deeper sacredness in the daily work of dishwashing and diaper changing or go nuts. Many people believe that there was once a time—a matriarchal age—when these "housewifely" tasks of maintaining the home and hearth were seen as the most sacred tasks of all. Our contemporary culture has certainly reversed that attitude. But even today, wherever women—and men along with them—have managed to succeed in discovering the sacred element in the creation of home and in the building and maintaining of a true hearth, there is Hestia, alive and well. Let me hasten to say, here, that I am not advocating the re-chaining of women to the kitchen sink. Far from it. I believe that true feminism is about freedom of choice. However, by ceasing to honor Hestia and devaluing the importance of hearth, home and child-rearing, our society has actually removed some of that choice by making many younger women ashamed of their secret wishes to stay home for a few years. And, of course, by making it increasingly hard for them to afford to, even if they want to.

Our world needs both visions, the masculine and the feminine. We need to soar and we need to plumb the depths, and wisdom lies in both directions. Just as in architecture, we need the inspiration of the awesome—as in the beautiful gothic cathedrals of Europe and modern marvels like the Sydney Opera House—we also need built environments which honor Hestia, places with a center, places which speak to us in Christopher Alexander's Pattern Language that I mentioned in Chapter 6, places built to suit the human heart. We need to go out, fly high, have adventures. And we need to come home again to the center.

In shamanic traditions, there are various directions in which to journey—up and out or down and in. For the elderwoman, both are necessary. Her way is often the way of gentleness and subtlety, caring and compassion, and yet she has the necessary far-seeing—the deep vision and detachment—to make her work and her words optimally effective. She may need the occasional trip up to the revolving restaurant to get a refreshing glimpse of the view and restore her perspective. But I believe the most crucial factor is probably the journey in. The wisdom acquired in the flickering firelight of her own inner hearth.

Hestia, that quiet, reflective goddess of the hearth, who breathes the sacred into everything, must now, in this third age of ours, be invited into every aspect of our lives. For without her, there isn't any "there" there.

BLOOD
fire as personal passion and family relationship

15

As I MENTIONED earlier, the guiding metaphor for my previous book was the ancient belief that the menstrual blood, when it is no longer required for the making of babies, transmutes into wisdom. In that book, I spoke also of the old woman who, once her bleeding ceases, no longer holds the mysterious power of which the male is so often deeply afraid, and is thus set free. In some cultures, her freedom from female blood rhythms brings her greater power. She is given status and power as an honorary man and entrusted with tribal secrets.[1] In others, her departure from the fertile cycle of childbearing and child-rearing renders her of no further consequence and she is left to her own devices:

> An enemy would no more consider it worthwhile attacking
> her than killing a worthless animal [sic]. Therefore she
> need not fear the anger of ancestors, the malevolence of
> evil spirits nor indeed infection by disease. She can
> undertake the most hazardous tasks with equanimity.[2]

In our present-day culture, where most of us can expect to live another twenty or thirty years beyond menopause, we have a third option which incorporates all the freedoms of these other two with none of the disadvantages. This is to grow into an elderwoman.

The elderwoman in our own culture has no need to be initiated into the tribal secrets of the men, for she herself is trustee of far more ancient and fundamental tribal secrets than they are. In fact, her key task is to see that these secrets are retaught to them so that life on Earth comes into balance and regains its health before it is too late to save it.

It makes no difference how or where she chooses to do this reteaching. It is the same task, whether she is lobbying a politician, giving a lecture, writing a poem or telling stories to a grandchild.

The elderwoman's family connections maintain her influence at home, while her newfound freedoms—from paid work, from childcare, from worrying about what others think—mean she can operate anywhere she chooses. So she has two potential spheres of influence, personal and political. This chapter focuses mainly on the personal while the next deals with the social and political.

Blood, we say, is thicker than water. Although we may at times feel frustrated and even damaged by certain family relationships, they influence us crucially in two ways. One is our day-to-day dealings with relatives, the other is the way we were shaped by our families of origin

Regardless of how powerful the figures of our parents or other caretakers may have been, by the time we reach sixty, the scene will have changed, outwardly, at least. If our parents are still alive, they are probably by now more frail, more dependent. Role reversals may have taken place, with former caretakers now needing our care, sometimes on a daily basis. This is something which makes life particularly difficult for many women during their menopausal years. At the very time they are needing to withdraw into the menopausal cocoon, they may find themselves more in demand than ever. Though children have often left home, or at least have attained a degree of emotional and physical independence, elderly parents are starting to need more attention. And for those who have been later in having their own families, there may even be a combination of adolescent children and needy parents all clamoring at the same time—the worst time possible for someone whose hormonal fluctuations, mood swings and hot flashes are already creating internal havoc.

About the only thing we can say to women who are in this particular maelstrom of feelings, conflicting demands, inner confusion and weariness is "Hang in there—it *will* get better."

And it does. Unless we have offspring with special needs, by the time we reach seventy, most of us will have buried both of our parents and waved our children—if we have them—goodbye. For many, this time will come earlier. Much as we loved them all, much as we miss them, this can also be a wonderful sigh-with-relief time. A time when we can turn our attention fully to the twin tasks of the elderwoman, i.e. the inner journey of wholeness and the outer journey of being a wise elder. A time to enjoy any grandchildren or great-grandchildren we may now have—then hand them back at the end of the day.

For many of us, it is a time when solitude starts to become really important. Yet our relationships, particularly with kin and close friends, are increasingly precious to us after we leave the work world. So we may find these relationships going in two directions at the same time. On the one hand, there is an increasing detachment, and on the other, a deepening love and appreciation.

Feminist author Carolyn Heilbrun writes about this beautifully in *The Last Gift of Time: Life After Sixty*. She begins by describing how, when she was in her late sixties, she bought herself a house, despite the fact that she and her husband already owned one. Her husband understood. She knew that he understood her impulse to be less about house-buying than a yearning for solitude.

> *Solitude, late in life, is the temptation of the happily*
> *paired; to be alone if one has not been doomed to*
> *aloneness is a temptation so beguiling that it carries with it*
> *the guilt of adultery...*[3]

Nevertheless, it was not separation from her partner that she was seeking. In fact she welcomed him as her first guest. The new house was a concrete symbol of her selfhood, a place that was hers alone, to which she could retreat, away from family, friends, social expectations and the binding patterns and habits of the past. It was a symbol of her elderwoman freedom.

I was delighted to read her comments on relationships with her children and grandchildren, for her feelings exactly matched my own. Much as she adores the little ones, and enjoyed watching them grow, her greatest pleasure is in her own grown-up children. That is my experience also. I have found my ongoing dialogue with my now adult children both fascinating and inspirational. Watching one's own offspring meet the developmental challenges of their twenties, thirties and forties is every bit as fascinating as watching them move from milestone to milestone in their infancy and toddlerhood. When they reveal, in conversation, the depth of their understanding of the world and the insights they already have which may have taken me fifty laborious years to reach, I am awestruck. For me, as for Heilbrun,

...They are friends with an extra dimension of affection.[4]

Of course, as Heilbrun also acknowledges, there is yet another dimension to these relationships. No matter how hard we might have tried to be the perfect parent, there will inevitably be some lingering resentment somewhere inside our sons and daughters, some sense of old injustice or lack of understanding, however trivial this might now appear to have been, especially to us. Some innocent remark we make, if it carries even the tiniest tinge of judgment, might suddenly trigger off a totally unexpected response of anger, defensiveness or pain in this man or woman who was once our little boy or girl and at the mercy of our care, our rules and our worldview.

When this happens, it is all too easy to slip into a matching state of anger, defensiveness or pain ourselves. But before we do, better to take a deep breath, count to ten and stand by to discover something new instead. In my experience, these little moments of hurt and awkwardness, if carefully and non-defensively processed, can lead to deep insights and an even greater closeness. Unfinished business gets finished, old accounts are closed. Healing happens. We should welcome such moments rather than fearing them.

It is fascinating to be singing the other part in a duet we already know very well. For as we all know, we were shaped by the experiences of our own childhoods, and some of that old pain may still be with us. Furthermore, most of us will not have the advantage that our children have, which is the opportunity to process issues with our mothers or fathers. Even while our own parents were alive, they were unlikely to have been open to such things, being of an older and less psychologically literate generation. Possibly, we kept trying anyway. But when they are gone, we may feel that the last opportunity to close outstanding accounts with them has gone also.

This is not so. All the clearing I needed to do with my own father has been done since his death, and from all my years of clinical practice I know this to be true for many. Much successful work on the healing of relationships is done in this way, without the other person physically present.

There are many ways of doing it. The Gestalt technique of sitting the absent person in an empty chair, speaking your feelings to him or her and listening for—or even acting out—the response is a very effective tool, as is the use of letters. An exercise I have often suggested to people is this. Write a not-for-posting letter to the other person. Then write two letters to yourself. One is the response you would realistically expect to receive from the other person. The other is the response you would *like* to receive. Sit with all these a while. Finally, when you feel the emotions begin to ebb away, burn all three letters, visualizing the last remaining shreds of pain being borne away on the rising smoke. Then relax into a meditation, allowing all emotion to subside completely and healing to fill all the spaces.

While the former situation—the arising of unfinished business with our own offspring—happens only to those of us who have borne and/or raised children, the latter happens to us all. Our unfinished business with our own original families may erupt in numerous different ways, the most common of which is probably finding ourselves in conflict with people whose attributes are similar to theirs. An honest examination of our own feelings may then lead us to a recognition of some old, familiar pattern in our lives. ("This is just the way I used to feel when my father chewed my butt for bringing home a lousy school report...")

Those of us who have paid attention to the processes of menopause will have found that most of our important bits of unfinished emotional business will have come around again during this chaotic period of our lives and we shall have worked on them. By the time we get to our sixties, however, there seems to be a new mellowness to all this. The hurts remaining within us start to be bathed, now, by a sweet compassion for the whole human predicament. The ability, as we move into elderhood, to keep our eyes more and more on the "Big Picture"—like the astronaut who could see more and more of his home planet as the journey progressed— brings with it not only a more passionate caring about issues but also a greater compassion for all whom we judge in the wrong. It is an interesting paradox.

So for the elderwoman, who has done her personal inner work, there is less and less personal angst. In its place comes a sense of sureness and a sense of harvest. From her sureness, she now speaks out with confidence. And the harvest is both her wisdom and her deepening pleasure in life itself. It is the achievement of greater detachment from the cares and woes of the world and the personal troubles of others, plus her increasing ability to show compassion.

One of my daughters said to me last year that she finds it easier to tell me her problems nowadays because I no longer take them on board the way I used to when I was younger. She derives great comfort from the fact that I can now remain detached and caring at the same time. In turn, that makes it easier for her to hear any suggestions I might make, without the old filters of defensiveness. We have moved far beyond the old mother–daughter roles into the "friendship with the extra dimension of affection." It feels great.

It is probably for the same reason that many young people find it easier to confide in their grandparents than in their parents. This attribute of detached compassion is, more than anything else, the hallmark of the elder.

I have spoken of passion in terms of our depth of caring about people and issues, and I have talked a lot about compassion. But you may be wondering, what of sexual passion? What of love affairs, intimate relationships, new friendships?

One of the fascinating things about growing old is that as we age we become more and more who we truly are. So as regards our sexuality, I suspect we vary hugely in the way it manifests in our third age.

Jean Shinoda Bolen, in her book *Goddesses in Everywoman*, showed how the various Greek goddesses could be seen as archetypal forces expressed through the different lives and personalities of women.[5] So, just as a Demeter-type mother will differ in her parenting style from an Artemis-type mother, we can probably guess that a Hestia-sort of grandmother will feel different to an Athena-ish one. Those of us for whom the Aphrodite archetype has been a dominant one will probably continue to enjoy a passionate sex life right into old age. A Hera-sort of personality, for whom marriage is the all-important theme, may have a greater need of a partner than, say a Hestia woman, for whom solitude is a key requirement, or an Artemis-type, who values freedom and autonomy over everything else. For a Demeter-type, sex is more about procreation than recreation, so its importance to her may well diminish after menopause.

However, as Bolen points out, these archetypal influences move back and forth throughout our lives, making prediction difficult, but outcomes interesting. Bolen, herself an elderwoman now, has since written more extensively on how these archetypes manifest in us in our third age. Her follow-on volume *Goddesses in Older Women* includes not only the Greek goddesses but others drawn from different cultures to represent qualities the elderwoman may find in herself (such as Kwan-Yin for compassion).[6] It is a book I highly recommend.

The elderwoman, who is now free to be fully herself, may turn out to be sexier than ever. Or she may be thankful to let sex recede. The most important thing is not that she has or does not have sexual desire, but that her desire—or lack of it—will be fully authentic. All need to dissemble is now gone. She can be her true self, whatever that is.

If she lives with a partner, there may be need, now, to renegotiate some of the patterns of their shared life in order to accommodate her growing need for inward-turning time and new kinds of service. Or, if she is lucky, her partner, too, may be in a parallel process and their relationship will have mellowed in many delightful ways. In the unfortunate event that she finds herself taking care of a partner who has become ill or feeble, her time and energy may be severely circumscribed. But if she is able to bring every one of her elderwoman principles into action, she will probably find even this experience of intensive service becoming, like everything else, grist for the mill of her own spiritual development. Thus there will remain a deep joy in her life, despite the pain. For anyone in this position it is imperative to remember, also, that there must still be regular time off, time alone, time to recharge. Service must never become martyrdom, no matter how worthy the cause. The principle of respect must also apply to ourselves—and to our limitations.

For all except the exceedingly introverted among us, friendship remains important in our third age. After all these years, those few friends whose journeys have proceeded along similar lines to our own and who are still walking with us will have become as close as kin. They seem, by now, to be of the same blood as ourselves, so long have we been walking, talking and sharing. They are precious.

Those whose journeys have diverged widely may by now have dropped away. But in their place, new friendships arise. When they do, they seem to arise rapidly and with a sureness that is different from any of the tentative explorations of our earlier years. We find each other, we recognize each other and we go very deep, very fast. There is almost a freemasonry of elderhood. I have even experienced it in passing another woman in the street; a certain look, a certain knowing wisdom in the eyes, a special soul-to-soul smile that warms me for hours afterwards, like a hot water bottle for the heart.

For me, the great thing about making and maintaining an ever widening circle of friendships in my elder years is that nowadays friendship knows no barriers of geography. Thanks to e-mail, I can be in daily contact with the ordinary lives of friends and family members all over the globe, just as though they were living next door. My daughters and I call it "back-fencing," chatting about the little events of our day on e-mail, like neighbors meeting in the yard. To one Jungian friend I may tell a dream, and back comes a thought on what that dream might mean. With another I compare astrological forecasts for the week. I say a quick "hi" to my sister, tell another friend about a book I just read and hear about my daughter's day at work. The world is right here, on my desk.

Carolyn Heilbrun writes that she would like to ensure an e-mail connection for everyone over sixty-five. For the older and more sedentary we become, the more valuable this is for the maintenance of our links with family and friends no matter where they are.[7]

She might also have added that our use of the Internet enables our access to the political world and widens endlessly our possibilities for sharing our wisdom on a global scale. But that is for the next chapter.

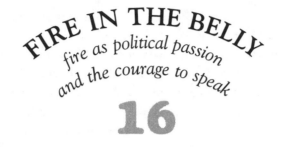

FIRE IN THE BELLY
fire as political passion and the courage to speak

16

As I HAVE emphasized many times, throughout this book, the distinction between knowledge and wisdom is an important one. I did not always realize this. It took motherhood to start me thinking about it.

When I was expecting my first child, I read as much as I could on the subject of pregnancy, birth and breast-feeding. When the baby was born, I bought a copy of Dr. Benjamin Spock's classic, *Baby and Child Care*, to find out how to do parenting. Later, unsatisfied with that alone, I began to ransack the library for everything I could find on the subject of child psychology, child guidance, etc. I figured that if I consulted the experts I would know how to do it right, and be able to raise perfect children. (Yes, I know. It makes me laugh too—and blush with embarrassment for my own naïveté.) To my astonishment, I discovered that there are as many theories as there are experts. And many of the so-called experts disagree completely.

It began to dawn on me, then, that perhaps my own thoughts and ideas on the subject had some value too. After all, if even the experts could not agree, perhaps there was room for personal research, intuition, instinct, figuring things out for myself? This may have been my first inkling of the fact that knowledge and wisdom are two different things. It was, I now suspect, the first time in my life that I really began to value my own internal wisdom as much as I valued the knowledge I could glean from libraries, classes and talking to other people.

Twenty years later, I came across a work entitled *Women's Ways of Knowing* by Mary Field Belenky and her team of associates, who did a series of in-depth interviews over several years in an attempt to find out how women acquire and convey their knowledge of the world, both in formal and in informal settings. The interview subjects varied in their educational experience, age, ethnicity and economic background.[1]

These researchers discovered firstly, as other researchers into gender differences in psychology had also found, that women usually approach life from a position of relationship and connection to those around them, whereas men tend to operate from a position of separation and autonomy. Secondly, they discovered certain key differences within their study group. They found that some women learn by passively receiving knowledge handed to them by "authorities" (as I had been attempting to do with the child psychology books) and others rely more on the use of their own intuitive wisdom. Lots of us, like me, rely on the former method in our younger years and then discover our own inner sources later on. We can imagine what might happen if one were to rely totally on either method alone. A complete and lifelong reliance on received wisdom will create a person who cannot think for herself and is thus a puppet in the hands of those who would control her. ("It must be OK... because I read it in the paper... because the Government knows what it is doing... because my mother/husband/boss/supervisor told me it was.")

Total reliance on our own inner processes, on the other hand, without some kind of reality check with the outside world, can lead, if we are not careful, to an insubstantial kind of flakiness which can make it difficult to live a competent and fully grounded life. ("It must be OK because I trust my guidance/the angels/the tea leaves/the stars/this discarnate entity, Fred, who I've been channeling...")

The mark of a fully mature woman, these authors conclude, is the ability to integrate these two ways of knowing. The results of this integration, field-tested in day-to-day experience, become true wisdom.

What we do with that wisdom, however, depends on many things. It depends, first of all, on individual character. What sort of people are we?

As James Hillman has pointed out, despite the many changes we go through as we grow and evolve as people, there is a basic "usness" which is always present. In *The Force of Character*, Hillman uses the delightful metaphor of a darned sock. No matter how many times it is darned, nor how much of the original wool has been replaced by the darning—theoretically even up to 100 percent of it—it is still the same sock. Regardless of the fact that almost all of our body's cells are continually dying and being renewed, so that every few years we are virtually made of different material, we remain absolutely and recognizably ourselves.[2]

The older we get, the more evident that becomes. Character seems to deepen with age, like the laughter lines around our eyes. What needs to go along with that deepening is a corresponding inner acceptance that we are who we are. If it feels comfortable to stand up and shout from a soapbox about the things we see wrong with the world, then the freedom we feel as elderwomen gives us the go-ahead to do it, and to hell with anyone who disapproves. But if preaching from a soapbox fills us with horror, and that type of public expression of our beliefs is just not our way, then it would be doing violence to ourselves to try and make ourselves do it.

I want to stress this freedom to you strongly, for in my revealing to you of some of my own more exuberant antics, I fear you may imagine me to be issuing a prescription for the elderwoman's life which is based on *my* particular character. And this is not my intention. If there is one thing I have learned from my own grandmother, it is that one quiet word or silent smile, correctly placed, is just as powerful as a torrent of words. Both the gentle harp and the noisy kettledrum make their unique contributions to the orchestra. You do not have to be an activist to be an activist, if you see what I mean. Every third-age woman within whom that elderwoman sense has ripened and developed is an activist of sorts. Each one does activism in her own unique way, as determined by her character and preferences.

My grandmother's direct influence upon the world was very slight. She moved mostly in family and church circles and rarely traveled beyond her home town. Yet her influence was strong. It was strong in that her little wise sayings have passed down through several generations. And it was strong in that she lived her values so truly and with such integrity in her own life that she was like a beacon to the people around her and the memory of her has lived on in others, including me.

So our individual characters, along with other factors—opportunities, abilities and so on—will determine the exact manner in which our wisdom is transmitted. It may be through art or poetry, through music or craft. It may be through speaking out, writing letters, marching in demonstrations. It may be reflected in the things we join, the causes to which we donate, the ways we spend our time. It may be transmitted by look or gesture, a few words here or there, a comforting touch, a well-chosen card. It may be that we simply, like my grandmother, live out our values with integrity and become models for those around us. There are as many ways of being an elderwomen as there are elderwomen to experiment with them.

The other key factor which influences us to find ways of channeling our own collected wisdom is the increasing confidence that our wisdom is worth channeling. Thirty-five years after my discovery that the experts did not agree, something else became suddenly clear to me, which is that the so-called experts are often completely wrong anyway. Remember how a certain pharmaceutical company's experts convinced everyone that there was no proof of the relationship between thalidomide and birth malformations? Remember how the tobacco companies produced whole teams of experts to explain that there was no link between smoking and disease? Remember how we were assured by experts that DDT was perfectly harmless? How the British Government experts assured the populace that humans were safe from mad cow disease? Many such reassurances cost lives.

They are still at it. Expert scientists in the pay of the transnational chemical companies insist that there are no dangers in bio-engineering. Genetically engineered (GE) soybeans were passed by the FDA as being substantially equivalent to non-GE soybeans even though many of the FDA's own scientists had written reports to the contrary. One of the worrisome aspects of genetic engineering—the possibility of what is known as horizontal gene transfer taking place—was dismissed by the experts. It cannot happen, they said. Within a couple of years, experiments with honeybees proved beyond doubt that it could—and had—happened. Nevertheless, the experts continued to say it could not happen, and dismissed the fears around it as foolish.

My realization, as a young mother, that my own inner wisdom was of equal—or greater—value to me than the advice of the experts fired me with confidence. So again as an elderwoman, the sudden dawning of the fact that we, not "they," are the real experts is the one thing which, more than any other, has served to light my inner fire. It is from that deep and sure knowing that I now find myself marching forth, sword in hand, to fight in whatever ways I can for those things in which I most passionately believe.

I know for certain that I am not alone. There is a rise of indignation in the elderwoman whose ranks are forming now. We have got it that we have just as much authority as anyone else—in fact, more—in terms of knowing what is right. We are it. We are the elders, the far-seers. When this really hits you, it is an amazing realization!

I have noticed that the fire of political passion that burns in me today is very different in quality from the one which burned in my youth. Though I was unaware of it at the time, for the first thirty years of my life, whatever political opinions I had were all held in my head. Like many other young people of my generation, I went through phases of political posturing, but now, when I look back, I can see that it was all a part of that trial-and-error thing we call identity formation, like the year I bought my first duffel coat and desert boots and walked around with a Communist Party newspaper under my arm and an earnest expression on my face, or sat in coffee shops discussing revolution with equally earnest, similarly dressed young men. We all chain smoked, back then, and listened to Russian orchestras on the short wave radio playing wobbly versions of "The East is Red" in between propaganda messages (of which we understood not one word, of course, since they were all in Russian. But they sounded right). And what I was really interested in, though I could never have admitted it at the time, was the young men themselves and which of them might be the most likely to fancy me.

It took motherhood to put me in touch with real political action. And I don't mean party political either. I mean political in the true grassroots sense of the word.

Our local authority announced that it would be spraying dieldrin, a deadly poison, to kill fruit flies all around our neighborhood. My baby was a few months old. I thought about her little lungs, breathing in that deadly vapor and suddenly I was transformed into a she-tiger. For the first time, politics were in my gut and in my heart, and no longer in my head. At the same time, from the front doors of all my neighbors, an army of she-tigers—and he-tigers—came pouring out. Many meetings, demonstrations, and angry shouting matches later, the spraying program was stopped. We had won. My first political victory. It tasted sweet.

Then came the Vietnam War. High drama. Marching through the streets in a mighty throng, singing, chanting, waving banners. The incredible feeling of sitting in absolute silence with several thousand other people, right in the middle of a city intersection, as the roll of young men's names was slowly read out—young men killed in their prime by a senseless, crazy war.

There were anti-nuclear marches, political rallies—so many causes, so many reasons for despair and also for solidarity, for the linking of arms, the shedding of tears and the heightened intensity of shared passion.

But now?

The elderwoman's passion, informed as it is by her understanding of the Bigger Picture, a lifetime of experience and a deeper insight into human nature, is always accompanied by its wise sister—compassion, which, in some ways, makes things all the harder.

I once listened in on a talk given by psychologist Joseph Chilton Pearce to a group of Siddha Yoga devotees, disciples of the late Baba Muktananda, who had died some months previously. Pearce, himself a devotee, described how he had boasted to another disciple about the passionate speech he had recently given, all about the horrors of war, and denouncing the Pentagon. Baba, he said, would have been proud of him. The other, more seasoned disciple shook his head. "No," he said. "You don't understand. You see, Baba loves the Pentagon." With his panoramic view of the world and humankind, the Yoga sage knew that everything had a place in the scheme of things—even war and the Pentagon. So although Baba almost certainly hoped for a world beyond war, his judgment of society and its feeble structures was encompassed by compassion. Love thine enemies. This was Christ's message also.

So for the elderwoman, no matter how strong her idealism, no matter how angry and despairing she may become about the despoliation of the world or how judgmental she may feel of those she is disposed to blame, there is always a level at which she also feels compassion, not only for those she sees as victims but for those she sees as the oppressors also. It is not that she approves their actions. And at the political or personal level, she may be opposing those actions with every means at her disposal. But at a deeper, spiritual level, she also has compassion. The two are not mutually exclusive.

Vietnamese Buddhist monk, Thic Nhat Hanh has written a beautiful poem on this entitled "Please Call Me By My True Names." He wrote it after receiving a letter about a twelve-year-old refugee girl who threw herself into the sea and drowned because she had been raped by a sea pirate. It would be easy, he explained, to feel like shooting the pirate. But he knew that if he had been born in the same village as the pirate and experienced the same life, he may well have grown up to be a pirate instead of a monk.[3] Compassion opens the door of the heart so wide that we can put ourselves in the place of everyone. Sometimes, as in the case of the sea pirate, it has to be a very big and difficult stretch.

So our passion and our compassion belong together. I have changed the order so that they can sit next to each other of our list of elderwoman principles.

• simplicity • deep vision • passion • compassion • non-attachment • Earth-centeredness • comfort • connectedness • respect • creativity • delight • lightness • enoughness • heart-listening • peace and quiet •

The fire that burns in the elderwoman burns in her belly, in that deep center of her that now truly knows the extent of her own authority and has, for the first time, the courage to speak her own truth in an authoritative way, regardless of the so-called experts, most of whom, unfortunately, seem better at ax-grinding than they are at wisdom. It also burns in her heart, in a compassion as wide as the world and as deep as the ocean—not always an easy mix of fires to have going on inside one's aging body.

One of Belenky's findings, in her study of the ways in which women acquire and convey knowledge of their world, was that some women— often from the ranks of the poor and disadvantaged—are never able to incorporate the information they receive from outside into their own understanding of the world.[4] And neither are they able to access their own inner wisdom. They are thus condemned to silence. So those of us who are fortunate enough to be able to make our voices heard must also speak out on behalf of our silent sisters.

I am fond of quoting Florida Scott-Maxwell who, writing in her eighties about the passions which burned in her, remarked, "All this is very tiring, but love at any age takes all you've got."[5] She might have added "And to add compassion, takes more than you ever thought you had!"

But hey, what would you rather do? Be an elderwoman, with all the pain, courage and growth which that entails, or while away your time playing bingo and regretting a half-lived life? I know *my* choice.

TAKING THE RISK
personal iconoclasm, the fiery and outrageous elderwoman

17

IN PREVIOUS chapters, we have looked at fire as the hearth—the center, or focus, of our lives and landscapes—and fire as passion, both personal and political. Now I want to turn to another attribute of fire, which is its capacity to transform.

We are made of fire. Our entire Universe began fifteen billion years ago, as a great fireball. After another billion years, the galaxies formed— one hundred million of them, including our own Milky Way. And from there, five billion years ago, our sun was born, and in its turn gave birth to life. All life on Earth, all growth, remains totally dependent on that ball of fire in the sky, our daily reminder of the power and heat of the original fireball.[1]

There is nothing in existence which was not once part of the fireball. All we are was ever present. Nothing has been lost, nothing added. So what we are today, all of us, is simply a part of that fireball, in its ceaseless movement toward greater and greater complexity. Fire is everything. Fire, as the element called *pitta* in the Ayurvedic medical system, is an important ingredient of our human constitutions.[2]

Heat is a vital factor in the process of composting, or turning dead matter into soil. When you first build a compost heap, it heats up, beginning the process of transformation.

When I first began experiencing the hot flashes of menopause, I immediately thought of them as the beginning of a transformational process which was happening right within my own body and psyche. With each one, I visualized myself changing, transforming, as a caterpillar transforms into a butterfly. This time it was not the garden waste, the kitchen scraps and last fall's dead leaves which were being composted, it was me. I did not know what it would be like to emerge at the other end of this menopausal process, but I intuitively knew that the process was profoundly transformational. I knew that I would arise from it renewed, just as the phoenix arises from the ashes of the fire. The same me would come forth, but maybe with different ideas, different preoccupations, different passions.

Post-menopausal passion seems to burn as a finer, keener flame than the passions of our earlier days. It is a passion which fills whatever work we do with radiant energy, for now there is nothing held back. We no longer fear censure. We are beyond caring what other people think. Like the "worthless" old woman I spoke of in Chapter 15, we pose no apparent threat to anyone, and that same cloak of invisibility provides our immunity. So we can flit unnoticed through the structures of our society, taking up our sniper positions. We can speak out, stand up for what we believe in, in whatever way we choose, and if we get reproachful looks we simply laugh—the delighted cackle of the crone.

One of the most rewarding aspects of being old—and one which makes many an elderwoman chuckle with delight—is the permission we now feel to be "outrageous."

When Jenny Joseph's poem *Warning* first came out, with the immortal line: *"When I am an old woman I shall wear purple."*, it was passed around from woman to woman, like a talisman. Everyone who read it smiled in instant recognition of the impulse within herself to break free in her old age and be her ultimate, outrageous self. Not surprisingly, given the degree of resonance it created, the poem became better and better known as time went on, eventually providing the title for a book.[3]

There is a whole literature around this principle of outrageousness in elderly women, ranging from the mythical story of Baubo, the old woman who shocked the grieving Greek goddess Demeter into laughter by exposing her ancient genitals, to modern studies in anthropology and social psychology and now, several books for the popular market, such as *Be an Outrageous Older Woman*.[4]

What is defined by some as outrageous is seen by others as a celebration of creativity and freedom. After a lifetime of conforming to the norms of "ladylike" or other "appropriate" behavior, the post-menopausal woman can at last be whoever and whatever she likes. Far from mourning our exclusion from old forms of security, we find ourselves, to our great surprise, celebrating our opportunities for new creativity.

One of the things I have enjoyed most about getting old is breaking free of what Naomi Wolf calls "The media construction of the 'sin of aging.'"[5] As Wolf so incisively points out, the whole so-called beauty industry is a monster. In its endless push for bigger and better profits, it dominates the lives of women, leaving not only stress and maxed out credit cards in its wake but anorexia and even suicide. We can never be beautiful enough to satisfy this greedy beast, for it knows that if we were to achieve perfection, we would stop buying, and then it would starve.

There are deep-seated reasons why we find it so difficult to avoid hooking into all of this. If we are heterosexual females, one of the strongest imperatives of our biology is to make ourselves attractive to the male of our species. Regardless of our own preferences, it is what *he* goes for that we go for. It is what he likes to see that we parade before his eyes, whether consciously or not. We can no more help ourselves from doing this, in some degree, than a female baboon can stop her backside from becoming a huge, swollen, brightly-colored advertisement for sex whenever her estrogen is high.

Despite the fact that our rational minds tell us that high-heeled shoes are bad for our posture and ruinous to our feet, that sunbathing may give us cancer, that advertising exploits us and the beauty industry is a monster feeding on our checkbooks, for the majority of us the siren call of our biology cannot be entirely blocked out.

It was already beginning to call me, way back in those far-off days when I begged Grandma to twist my hair into rags and make ringlets. By the time I was fifteen, the call had become a roar. I was obedient to that demanding roar all through my teens, twenties, thirties and forties, just like most other women I know.

As I mentioned in Chapter 2, menopause is a bit like being handed not just one challenge but a folder of separate challenges, each of which must be completed before we can graduate. One of them is the challenge that, for many women, is the hardest; I call it "fading roses." It is the challenge of watching our youthful petals fall and knowing that although we may fight and fight to preserve them, in the end there are only two options. One is to finish up—after repeated visits to the cosmetic surgeon—wearing a tight and characterless mask, a gruesome parody of our own youthful face. The other is to relax and drop out of the game altogether.

Letting go can be scary. It can be depressing. There were several years during which I would catch sight of myself, from time to time, in a bus window or the unforgiving, all-revealing mirror of a store fitting room and wonder, with horror, "Who is that old woman? Surely that cannot be me?"

People no longer said, "Oh you look so young." They started saying, "Oh you are looking so much like your mother these days." After a while, I became used to it. I resigned myself to the fact that I no longer looked younger than my years.

I am not sure, now, exactly when the next change happened. I think it was a gradual thing, over several years. All I know is that the old biological siren call disappeared. In its place, was a beautiful, comforting silence. Now, at last, I could be me. I could look however I wanted to look, wear whatever I felt like wearing, not out of any sense of defiance but simply out of the sensuous pleasure of dressing for comfort and pleasing myself. If I felt sexy, I could be outrageously, ridiculously sexy, like Baubo, in honor of all the things my body had seen and done and felt over a long lifetime. If I did not feel sexy at all, I could be celibate, and be comfortable with my celibacy. It was a feeling of freedom and of celebration. The celebration of my whole self. I was free of the beast, at last. I had come home to myself. Home safe.

I recall reading, many years ago, Barbara McDonald and Cynthia Rich's pioneering work, *Look Me in the Eye*,[6] and resonating with their sense of outrage at the way society renders old women invisible. Those authors were particularly incensed that they saw this same process occurring even within the ranks of lesbian women, who one would expect to be most supportive of their elderly sisters. I felt for them. The word "ageism" entered my vocabulary at that point, alongside sexism and racism, as a thing to be deplored.

In those days, however, my own response of outrage was for the most part an intellectual one. Some years later, while researching for my book on menopause, I re-read their book. Once again I felt the outrage, but this time it was personal, powered by my own experience of creeping invisibility and the inexorable falling of my own petals.

The third time I read it, a new feeling had crept in. By now, I was completely at peace with the concept of being old, and the elderwoman spirit was rising in me. The phoenix was emerging from the transforming fire. Now, having ceased to care that people had mostly stopped saying, when they heard my age, "Oh you don't look *nearly* as old as that!" I suddenly started hoping they would say it again. For I had thought up a neat response. The first time I tried it out, it worked beautifully. I was reminiscing with distant relative of mine, who I had not seen for years. "Let me see, how old are you now?" she asked me.

"Sixty-four," I answered.

"Oh goodness me, you certainly don't look it," she said.

"Well that's a pity," I said. "I was rather hoping I did. I like being old."

Her eyes widened in astonishment. She then got a short lecture on ageism.

My next victim was a very polite man who lives not far from me. We are acquaintances, rather than friends. I cannot remember how we came to be discussing age, but I told him mine.

"Oh my dear, you don't look nearly that old," he said, obviously trying to give me a compliment.

I looked him straight in the eye. "So if I did, would you find me ugly, then?" I asked innocently.

Poor man. He went all red and flustered. He got my mini-lecture on ageism too.

When Baubo spread her legs to make Demeter laugh, the humor arose, not from the ancient vulva she displayed, but from the paradox. When someone who is meant to fade into the invisibility of old age suddenly pops up and says "Boo!" at the most unlikely moment, the effect is electrifying. So if the inner aspect of our outrageousness is the celebratory aspect—our delight in pleasing ourselves—the outer aspect is our ability to shock other people awake. We may do this to make a political point, as I was making to these two people about ageism, or we may do it simply because it is, quite frankly, a lot of fun. We get a kick out of it in the same way that a little child gets a kick out of making grownups jump.

The child's giggle of delight and the crone's cackle have a lot in common. And the first time we hear that cackle rising in our throats we know that old age is going to be, among other things, quite a joyride. Like pots, we have been in the fire. And now we are baked hard and strong. Strange, unpredictable pots—crackpots, maybe—wearing what we like, eating what we like, getting up and going to bed when we feel like it, pouring our passions into this or that, celebrating, pontificating, laughing, meddling, interfering, being difficult, wearing purple, spitting, refusing to fit into boxes any longer, and being generally outrageous. In other words, enjoying ourselves hugely in the late afternoon sun.

It is not the outrageousness itself which is the underlying principle here, of course, for there are some elderwomen who rarely, if ever, step outside the norms of their group. The point is not that they exhibit the quality of outrageousness but that they now have the potential to do so. Since such a quality arises from the freedom to be completely oneself at last, the principle which underpins it—and a key one on our list—is authenticity. Now, more than ever before, we truly are who we are.

• simplicity • deep vision • passion • compassion • non-attachment • Earth-centeredness • comfort • connectedness • respect • creativity • delight • lightness • enoughness • heart-listening • peace and quiet • authenticity •

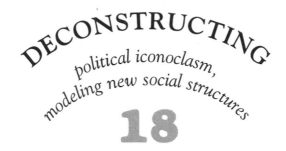

DECONSTRUCTING
political iconoclasm, modeling new social structures

18

FIRE HAS the power to destroy, cleanse and purify. Phoenix-like, the elderwoman in ourselves arises when that which is no longer needed has been destroyed.

Although this whole notion of destruction sounds violent and forceful, in practice the removal of those aspects of our lives which are no longer appropriate for us in old age seems to happen gradually, over a period of years. The unused lipstick lies in the corner of the drawer, the high-heeled shoes gather dust for a long, long time in the bottom of the closet. After decades of listening to certain favorite kinds of music, I now find those tapes remaining unplayed and I am drawn to different sounds and rhythms. Activities I used to relish, no longer hold a thrill, while others, recently discovered, capture my mind and heart. And when I look in the familiar corners of my mind for inspiration, it is no longer forthcoming. It arises, instead from new places, formerly unknown to me. So it is not a sudden destruction we are speaking of here, but rather a slow and gentle process of deconstruction of our old selves. This fire is a low, steady burn, rather than a leaping flame.

If we have gone through our menopausal years with an attitude of inner attention, and remained fully aware of our process, this deconstructing of our former selves may be experienced as a gentle dropping-off of what is now obsolete in our lives, like leaves falling off the tree (although a friend of mine whose physical menopause was triggered by surgery once told me that for her that loss of leaves felt more like the result of a gale. Like induced labor, her process was shorter, sharper and steeper).

Interestingly enough, deconstruction was also a popular theme in late-twentieth century philosophy. The sophisticated pundits of postmodern academia amused themselves by taking an ax to many of the smug certainties of the Western philosophical tradition and smashing them. The old icons we had worshipped were swept away. Everything was now seen as relative. There was no intrinsic meaning in anything any more.

This was reflected in the art of the times. Images, like the empty bean cans of Andy Warhol, stripped of all connection to deeper, more mystical truths, bereft of any redemptive possibility, merely mirrored for us the banality of life in the postmodern consumer society.

When we have smashed the old icons of a culture, the yearning for certainty—any structures being better than none—can easily lead to a situation where we settle for much less than we need or deserve; one where we put up new structures in a hurry, and then become content to stay with those, like DIY builders living permanently in the shed because we have run out of money and/or energy to build the house.

Historically, we have smashed many of the ancient systems which did not serve us well—the feudal system, for instance. But we did not necessarily create anything better.

When people became busy outside their homes and there was no time to cook a proper meal, fast food came on the scene. Now there are many who live on fast food alone. Thus the quality of our national diet goes steadily down. The old ways were smashed and the new replacement is of inferior quality. It happens over and over again, in myriad ways.

For many people who are dismayed by the loss of the value system they were brought up with as children, the response has been to turn for comfort to the simplistic, carved-in-stone certainties of fundamentalist religion. Like frightened teenagers running home to childhood, they flee from the need to think for themselves and to face all the difficulties and paradoxes out there in the world. Our science, moving much too fast for our ethics, hands out moral brain teasers every day: frozen embryos, organ transplants, cloning. These are hard things to think about; easier, surely, to parcel it all up and hand it to the preacher to sort out.

For others, the response to the rapid meltdown of the world they thought they knew is a tendency to over-idealize life in the "old days." These people, instead of looking forward, will try to persuade everyone that we should go back. Back to "family values," which is often shorthand for saying that women should lose the equal rights they have fought—and are still fighting—for and be forced into domesticity whether it is their choice or not, that men and women should be only heterosexual, that divorce is wrong, and so on.

To be sure, there are many things about the past that we have lost and need to rediscover. The wisdom of old farming methods, which preserved the fertility of the soil without chemicals; the nutritional value and superior flavor of wholegrain bread ground with stone instead of steel and baked in traditional ovens; the pleasure, comfort and healthiness of natural materials in our houses and clothes instead of the toxic hazards of today. But we need to pick and choose. Too often, we romanticize the past. We forget the downside of life in the old days, the fleas in the horsehair mattresses, the unhealthy cholesterol load in the "bread and dripping," the cruelty of bear-baiting, the inhumanity of slavery, the evils of workhouse and asylum. We need to go forward, not back. And the only sure way to go forward is to look at ourselves, at our needs, at what it is to be a human being and to work out, for ourselves, the optimum way to live, to live long, in health, harmony and accord with other creatures in the web of life.

So where deconstruction has paved the way for new beginnings, there is the everpresent danger of the space being taken up either by fundamentalism of many kinds or by a romantic, impractical sentimentality. In order to avoid these twin dangers, we have to do lots of thinking.

Our popular culture has been teaching us not to think. So it seems to me that one of the big ways in which each one of us elderwomen can begin to make a real difference in the world is simply by virtue of thinking. Most of the people scurrying around in the work world are too busy to think. Either their noses are too close to the coal face to see the overall shape of the seam, or they are too weary and stressed out to do more than watch TV till bedtime. Or if they are paid to think, they are also paid not to say or print what they really think—unless it results in profits for someone. Elders, on the other hand, have both time and perspective. We have vision and perception. And we have wisdom to bring to bear.

The elderwoman's remit is not an easy one. However, she has an advantage that few others have. The personal experience of deconstruction which she has lived through to arrive at old age has given her the very tool she needs in order to make sense of what is happening in the world. That is the ability to start again from scratch, keeping the best of the old and creating something new and wonderful with it. That very process which she is living is also the process our contemporary world is going through right now. The challenge she has faced is the selfsame challenge facing our contemporary society on a large scale. At a personal level, the challenge is this: do we stop thinking, turn on TV and become little old ladies, waiting to die? Or do we roll up our sleeves and become elderwomen? At the macro level, the challenge is: does our human society accept pollution, worsening inequality and injustice, global warming, the death of species, the gradual dimming out of life on Earth and just keep watching videos and spending money till everything is gone? Or do we look for a new way forward, instead?

There are more and more voices chiming in, lately, to affirm the latter choice. Crisis, as we know, can be a creative force in the lives of both individuals and societies, and we are facing crisis on a global scale. In addition to that, more and more of us are experiencing personal events which jolt us awake and make us start to think hard about the deeper questions of life. For, as Theodore Roszak has pointed out, with all the advances of modern medicine, particularly cardiac surgery, more and more people are entering their senior years by way of a medical crisis, which is, as he describes it:

> *a contemporary rite of passage that brings them face to face*
> *with their own mortality. The cultural and political importance*
> *of that increasingly commonplace experience should not be*
> *overlooked.*[1]

Roszak himself suffered just such a medical crisis. War and major surgery are two of the transformational opportunities in many men's lives. In the absence of initiatory rites of passage, for some these may be the only two opportunities. Either of these experiences is potentially transformational for women, too, of course. But even if we never experience either war or major surgery, we have menopause. And many of us have experienced pregnancy, birth and lactation. Women are used to major rearrangements of our bodies and emotions. So in many ways we are better prepared than men for this whole deconstruction/reconstruction business. We have all lived it.

A further important point which Roszak makes is that whether male or female, the first batch of elders of this twenty-first century have another defining characteristic. They are, he reminds us, the Flower Children grown old.

*Never before has an older generation been conversant with so
many divergent ideas and dissenting values. These are, after all,
people who, in their teens and twenties, lived through a time of
principled protest that seemed determined to subject every
orthodoxy, every institution, every received idea in our society to
critical enquiry.*[2]

Back when the maidens of the 1960s, with flowers in their hair, were
handing out daffodils on San Francisco's Haight Street and exhorting
everyone to make love instead of war, I was a decade ahead of them,
chronologically, and already well into the mother phase of my
development. Nevertheless, the liberalizing spirit of those times drifted
into my life too, encouraging me to think, re-appraise and evaluate the
lessons of my own youth. I was grateful to them for their wake-up calls.

Now it is my turn to call to them. Are you still there? Do you still care?
Will you come out again, with flowers in your gray hair and tell the world
what it needs to hear? Or have you tuned out, dumbed down, given up, sold
out, drowned in despair—or gone shopping instead? Somehow I don't think
so. I think you are already on your way, with a new message on your lips.

It is harder being young today. With so much general angst in the air,
many of our young people cannot help but respond with deep anxiety and
fear. As we know from psychiatry, free-floating fear in the individual can
lead to obsessive, ritualized behavior in an attempt to ward off danger and
regain a sense of control. Rituals, traditionally, are a way of warding off evil
spirits. The dysfunctional rituals we create as a result of our inability to
cope with modern life can make us crazy, for the demons we shrink from
nowadays are so large and so far beyond our individual control that we
become frantic in our attempts to keep them at bay.

This fear and powerlessness have created a whole range of
dysfunctional rituals and behaviors, from head-banging music and
vandalism to extreme, introverted obsession with computer games and the
virtual sex of Internet chat rooms. There is alcohol, of course, and more
types of drugs than ever before. Think, too, of the modern epidemic of
eating disorders, and of "shop till you drop," a compulsive scurrying from
purchase to purchase in a vain attempt to achieve an inner sense of OK-
ness. So you could say that as a culture we are suffering from obsessive-
compulsive disorder on a massive scale. Many of our young people have
been badly damaged by it, for example, the whole subculture of alienated

youngsters obsessed with suicide, creating their heroes from the ranks of the self-destroyed. I met many of them when I worked in the psychiatric ward of a large city hospital—fearful, despairing young wraiths, no longer able to imagine a life, longing only for darkness and release.

We cannot simply leave it up to younger people to fix the messed-up world we are bequeathing them. We have to get busy and fix it ourselves. Now.

There are, I am certain, just as many idealists among today's youth as there were in the 1960s. I have met a lot in my own wanderings. They deserve much praise, for against the background of today's mainstream materialist culture, youthful idealism has a harder time surviving. Today, it is the old, who have survived the ongoing epidemic of consumerism and come out of it with a new immunity, who are now our best hope for restoring order to an insane world. Roszak calls them "the New People". It is we who must take the responsibility. And it is responsibility that we must now add to our list, for that sense of shared responsibility for the health of our planet is one of the principles which marks us clearly out as elderwomen.

We have the experience, we have the wisdom, and we have the long view. We can look back a long way and forward a long way. So one of the elderwoman's tasks is to bear witness to the best things of the past and see that they are incorporated and integrated appropriately into a newly created future.

To accomplish this, she does not have to run for president. (Though, of course, she can if she feels like it. She might even get elected, one of these days.) The only thing necessary is for her to create a scale model of how she thinks the world should be. That scale model is her life. Then all she has to do is live it. As Gandhi once said, "Be the change you want to see in the world."

Quite simple, really, isn't it?

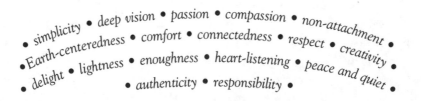

simplicity • deep vision • passion • compassion • non-attachment • Earth-centeredness • comfort • connectedness • respect • creativity • delight • lightness • enoughness • heart-listening • peace and quiet • authenticity • responsibility •

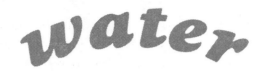

water

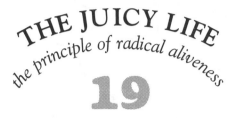

THE JUICY LIFE
the principle of radical aliveness
19

MOVING NOW to the water element, the first thing I want to consider is the way that the current of energy—"the juice"—runs through us now, in this third age. If we are beginning to feel it running through more strongly all the time, running so strongly that sometimes we worry that this river of life might burst our frail banks, then we are probably practicing radical aliveness. This, of all the elderwoman principles, is probably the most important. For in a sense, it contains all the others.

Radical aliveness is the art of saying "yes" to life; remaining fully open to all experience, whether pleasant or painful. It is the one thing—and the only thing—which can guarantee that our elderwoman years will be suffused with joy.

The idea, of course, is not new. The concept, in some form or another, has formed part of most of the world's great wisdom traditions for thousands of years, though it is more clearly discernible in some than in others. But the term itself—"radical aliveness"—is a fairly new one.

I love the term, and have used it ever since I first heard it, back in 1982. It was coined by Richard Moss, M.D., who gave up the practice of medicine in the 1970s to concentrate on matters of human consciousness. He used it to signify the full embrace of everything in one's own experience, rather than the judging of some parts of that experience as bad and some as good. It demands a willing acceptance of our pain and confusion and all the other negative feelings and an acknowledgment that they are as meaningful, relevant and full of learning potential as our joyful ones. In Richard's own words:

*The pain and uncertainty of life is not wrong. It is as right
as the joy and wonder of life. The only thing we can do is
knock upon all the doors. This is radical aliveness. We
begin to face the little death of yielding ourselves more fully
into life's immediacy.*[1]

According to this view, whether something that happens to us is
pleasant or unpleasant is irrelevant. Only aliveness matters. Opening,
saying "yes" to every experience that comes our way, creates a steady state
of joyfulness which shows up like a permanent watermark on every page of
our lives, regardless of what else is written there. It does not negate the
transient pains and pleasures which are part of each waking day. It
transcends them.

Thirty-seven years ago, when I was expecting my first child, I attended
classes to learn the techniques of natural childbirth. I wanted to give birth
in full awareness of the miracle that was happening to my body.

Marcelle, the physiotherapist who ran the classes was a vibrant,
energetic woman, who obviously loved her work and seemed to revel in
having her living room floor littered with pregnant women, lying there like
so many beached whales, practicing their breathing exercises under her
careful instruction.

Some were apprehensive. What would it be like, this new experience
of giving birth? Would it hurt? Could we cope? Yes, she said, we could.
Sure, there may be pain. There may also be rapture. It didn't really matter.
The important thing was to be totally there for it. Marcelle, in her
elderwoman wisdom, encouraged us to go forward to meet the unknown.
To say "yes" to whatever it turned out to be. To stay open to the experience.
"Life's for *living*, girls!" she would remind us.

Yes. I knew exactly what she meant. Life is for living. Not for
contracting away from. And that wise woman knew it. What we did not
know at the time, was that even as she cheered us on into our adventure,
Marcelle was facing a huge challenge of her own. None of us guessed she
was dying. One day, as she leaned over to adjust my position on the floor,
I caught sight of the edge of a mastectomy scar, and knew that she must
have had a brush with cancer. But it was still with her, and her life ended
just a few months after we had all given birth to our babies. I shall never
forget her zest for life and that brisk reminder to stay open to everything.

"Life's for *living*, girls." It was my first intimation of what radical aliveness was all about. I had no word for it then—just the memory of that voice, that cheery, no-nonsense injunction, "Life's for *living*."

It was many years later that I met Richard Moss and began to learn the full significance of radical aliveness. Through him, I came to learn that to live this way demands our full and complete involvement and willing immersion in every experience which life offers us, from the most tiny and insignificant, like watching an ant schlepping a breadcrumb, through the most ordinary and mundane, like brushing our teeth, to the most dramatic, like birth or death.

For someone who maintains this attitude, then whether an experience is judged good or bad, positive or negative does not matter. Painful things are still painful. In fact the pain may be sharper because one is more open to it. But it passes naturally, instead of lingering, and joy emerges again, like spring following winter. When we follow this philosophy, it is our degree of aliveness that counts—in everything. When we open to our experience, we expand. If we don't, we contract, and when we contract we shut down, like animals in shock. This not only makes us less available to others, it can also make us ill. Shutting down, if we are not careful, can become a habit, condemning us to the permanently contracted, fearful, escapist life of the walking dead. The habit of contraction arises from a deep feeling of insecurity, based in fear of death and of the unknown. Yet it is possible to go forward into the unknown—even the great unknown of death—with a zestful "yes!" rather than a fearful "no."

A grounded spirituality, which knows the human being to be an integral part of the fireball, forever part of the Earth, is a component of traditional elderwoman wisdom. So rather than trying to escape from our bodies, our lives or our daily experiences, our path to joy leads in the opposite direction. It leads more deeply into life, rather than away from it.

As we age, we are heading inexorably towards the earth. There is absolutely nothing we can do to prevent the inevitable fact that this body in and through which we live is destined for burial or burning. Like every other living thing, it will eventually return to the soil from which it sprang.

To resist that fact, to try vainly to lift ourselves up by our shoestrings and levitate away from this stark reality is not only patently ludicrous, but it also creates an inner block which prevents us from living fully. When the part of us which is trying to escape into the sky runs up against the part which is following its natural course towards the earth, it creates a logjam inside us. The current of life can no longer flow freely through us, sickness is likely and joy is diminished.

It follows, then, that what we need to ensure, in our later years, is our full and conscious alignment with this natural movement into the earth. After all, if we believe that our souls leave our bodies at death, it makes good sense to lower ourselves to the ground and relax, so that when the time comes for them to slip out, they can more comfortably and easily do so. And if those souls then move into another dimension, as I believe they do, it is not up in the sky somewhere, but right here, sharing this same space. If our earthly bodies are cells of the Earth's body, then surely our immortal souls are cells of the Earth's immortal soul too? This is home, after all. I don't think anyone is going anywhere else.

The older we get, the more likely we are to experience the stiffening and creaking and grumbling for which the elderly body is renowned. No matter how fit and healthy we are, inevitably our joints do wear, our bones get more fragile, our skin gets thinner. All the physiological processes slow down somewhat; healing takes a little longer.

The standard response to all this, in our culture, is to groan. "Oh I am getting old," we moan. "It's no fun getting old," someone said to me just the other day, and I heard several others agree with her, nodding their gray heads and pursing up their mouths in disapproval of this beastly aging process we are all being forced to suffer. "Getting old is absolutely *awful*," another woman said to me recently.

Well yes, sure it was nice to have a young, agile body and a future that felt endless. We were aging from the moment of our birth, of course, but no one said it was awful. We were impatient with childhood, eager to be sixteen, eighteen, twenty-one. It was exciting, being in our twenties, and thirty felt important. Then forty loomed and the first gray hairs, and the first beginnings of "awful." How sad and silly, to waste half our existence in futile condemnation of the very process—life—which brought it into being!

All this moaning and groaning about getting old is a bit like all the moaning and groaning I hear people doing about the weather. There is almost an indignation in it, as though they are being hard done by. As though things really shouldn't be that way. The fact is, they should. We need heat and cold, drought and flood, frost and rain, mist, strong winds, gentle breezes, hail and snow. We need them because they are part of the pattern of the world and the pattern is what keeps the world in balance. If the strong winds never blew, certain pollens would never spread, trees would not put down strong roots to brace themselves, the butterflies and birds who hitch rides on the air currents would never make their full journeys. Everything has its place in the pattern.

Creaking joints and failing energy have their part in the pattern too. All life is cyclic. It forever renews itself. Leaves have to fall off oak trees, old people have to age and die and new babies have to be born. As part of this whole, intricate, ever-cycling creation, we need to die, we need to age, we need to creak, to slow down, to feel ourselves growing old and feeble. It is part of being alive. And to feel it fully—to go with it, to align ourselves with its directionality, to watch in amazement that it is happening to us, too, just as at puberty we watched the miracle of our budding breasts, to rejoice in the wonder of it—that is all part of radical aliveness.

I remember when my hands first began to show the freckly blotches of aging that we call age spots. One day I looked at them and suddenly I could see my mother's hands, my grandmother's hands, the hands of my beloved Great-Aunt Jinnie. I stared in wonder at this transformation of the hands I had known since babyhood. Far from any desire to bleach the spots away, I looked at them almost reverently. It was as though I had been handed a passport. I was now a citizen of this same land from which my beloved elders came. I had joined them. I was one of them. As I stretched my hands out in front of me, I felt blessed and welcomed.

Developing this habit of saying yes to our experience means that we also say yes to all the experience of the world. So this kind of aliveness brings with it a tendency to have moments of almost unbearable sensitivity. We are no longer dull to horror or immune from the sadness of suffering. There are times when we feel so open, so vulnerable, so pulsatingly alive and so aware of everything, whether it be the scent of honeysuckle or the latest atrocity on the news, that it seems we could even die of it. At times like this, it is as though 1000 volts were coursing through a wire designed only for 110. And that, as I pointed out when we were discussing travel, is one of the reasons why we often need more rest and "time out" than younger people. We need to recover from those instances of almost unbearable responsiveness. You notice I said *almost* unbearable? For we can bear them—and we do. And like a workout at the gym, each one, although it may cause us to sweat a little, makes us fitter for the next.

• simplicity • deep vision • passion • compassion • non-attachment • Earth-centeredness • comfort • connectedness • respect • creativity • delight • lightness • enoughness • heart-listening • peace and quiet • authenticity • responsibility • radical aliveness •

Every moment contains the opportunity to say yes and also the potential for contraction. To stay open, to say yes, to walk forward with expectancy and to live deeply into all the experiences of our lives in this spirit of radical aliveness is the true elderwoman's way. And I really think it is the way to go. Life, after all, is for *living*. As juicily as possible. Right to the very last drop.

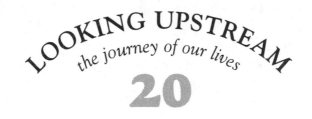

LOOKING UPSTREAM
the journey of our lives
20

So what does it take to become an elderwoman?

One thing I know for sure—it takes more than simply growing old. The elderwoman is not merely a woman who has reached her late fifties or sixties or seventies or beyond. Rather, she is one who has done so—or is now doing so—in a conscious way. She looks back over her life to see the paths she has traveled and looks forward to see how she might now contribute to her world. She has not only lived long enough to acquire both knowledge and wisdom but she knows and values the difference between them and she is prepared to go on acquiring the one and distilling the other.

The way I see it, knowledge is like a steadily growing heap of grain which we accumulate, kernel by kernel. Wisdom, on the other hand, is like malt. Just as malt is formed by fermentation—a result of natural processes like heat and time and the mysterious workings of yeasts—so is wisdom created by the application of our own life processes to the raw material of experience. Like that of malt, wisdom's nature also has a certain sweetness about it. If you don't quite get what I mean by that, try opening a really inspirational book and reading a paragraph or two. Notice the feeling it creates in you. Then look up a word in the dictionary or encyclopedia and note *that* feeling. And compare the two feelings. Each may contain a certain sense of satisfaction, but they are qualitatively different.

Just how do we extract the malt of wisdom from the grain of knowledge and experience? It is not easy to see how it is done, for it seems to happen by itself, somewhere deep inside us. Like digestion or the secretion of hormones, it is not under our conscious control. We merely experience the results of the process, as we proceed through our lives. Even as children, we are already beginning to create our store of wisdom and to display little nuggets of it from time to time. The sorts of things that cause parents to exclaim to each other, "Oh you'll never guess what she came out with today!" and note our cute sayings down proudly in journals, to be repeated back to us twenty years later.

It is in our third age, however, that the wisdom harvest begins in earnest. And one of the processes we begin to notice, in others and ourselves, is the one the gerontologists call "life review," in other words, spending time to look back over our own lives.

It is perhaps no accident that as we age, our long-term memory becomes sharper at the same time as our short-term memory is beginning to fray at the edges. Most elderly people can recall scenes of their childhood and youth with vivid clarity. It is almost as though we were programmed for reviewing our earlier lives when we get to the quieter, more sedentary days of old age and have some time to spare for it.

Remember the image I described in Chapter 9, of looking back along the path of a ritual procession and seeing it outlined in flares against the night sky? A life review is a bit like that. Except that we not only see the whole of the route we have taken, but we go back, in memory, to each section of the route, searching the ground for clues to our life's purpose. We look at what we have done, the goals we have achieved, the projects completed, the learning amassed. We search, too, for the lingering traces of abandoned dreams, for tasks left undone, paths not chosen, and we give a decent burial to those unmourned plans we find still languishing on life-support, waiting for us to see reason and pull the plug. Sure, it might have been a fantastic experience to walk the Inca trail all the way to Machu Picchu, and you promised yourself you would do it one day. But now? At seventy-five? Walking a strenuous path, at umpteen thousand feet, with your arthritic knees and your worsening emphysema? Er... maybe not.

For each one of us, the story will be different; the tasks of life review will vary widely, depending on who we are and have been. There is a sense, however, in which the human journey through life follows a common pattern.

Just as that now yellowed and dog-eared copy of Dr. Spock informed me about the all-important milestones of my children's development—

when to expect the first tooth, the first step, the first word—so have the milestones of developmental psychology provided a rough guide to the tasks of each life stage. The pioneer of human developmental studies, Erik Erikson, worked out, back in the 1940s, that each of us goes through a predictable sequence of stages, each of which has its central task.[1] In the same way that the central task of the adolescent is the formation of an individual identity and the task of the mature adult is to nurture and teach (the "generative" stage), the key task of this last stage of our lives is the development of a sense of what Erikson called "integrity."

Integrity—I really like that word. It gives a sense of wholeness, of integration of all the various parts of ourselves. For if we have been in the least aware of our own psychological processes over this past half-century-plus of living in these bodies, we must surely be aware by now that we are not simple unitary beings but more like a whole orchestra which may or may not play in harmony and which may or may not have an efficient conductor.

There have been many ways of conceptualizing this, ways which go in and out of fashion, disappear, reappear in new forms. We all know the Freudian concept of the ego (the orchestra's conductor), the id (the wild, unruly part of us that is bent on pleasure-seeking) and the superego (the stern parental conscience). In the 1960s, Eric Berne brought these ideas into the mainstream with his easy-to-understand writings about the "inner child" in its various forms (the "natural," free-spirited one and the "adapted" one we create to fit in with our family patterns), the "parent" in our heads and the rational, knowledge-seeking "adult."[2] The Italian psychologist, Roberto Assagioli, introduced Psychosynthesis, a way of looking at the whole cast of characters which lives within each one of us, resolving long-standing conflicts between them and understanding the purpose and value of each.[3] For each of these characters, no matter how problematical or self-destructive he or she may appear to be, is there for a purpose, in the same way that every instrument in the orchestra plays its vital part. The purpose may not be immediately apparent, but when it is, it will invariably be revealed as benign. When people act towards us in a misguided way but we know they have our best interests at heart, we can usually forgive them, and perhaps gently guide their actions in a better way. So it is with our inner cast of characters. Like a good film or theatre director, we aim to bring out the best in each of these characters and integrate their parts into a harmonious whole. This is the integrity project at its best. I recall a favorite example of this work in action.

One of my clients Joan, a social worker in her early fifties, after being introduced to the concept of Psychosynthesis, decided to investigate her own inner characters by writing them all into a one-act play. She did this at home, and brought it to me to read, the following week.

The action of her play took place in an old-fashioned English seaside guest house, where the various personalities who inhabited Joan's psyche were all together in the guest lounge, having afternoon tea and discussing their lives. Joan described each of them in the preamble, as she visualized them.

One character, a rather pale, thin, regal-looking woman in a blue dress, said nothing. Neither did she make any movement. All the other characters were buzzing about, pouring cups of tea, handing around cake and engaging in spirited dialogue, but this mysterious woman simply sat, staring straight ahead. Joan was really bothered by this woman. She called her "Lady Blue." She knew that this character was a part of herself that she despised. It was the part of her which sometimes spent whole days "veging out" in the chair, avoiding activity and other people, when there was a mountain of things to be done. Lady Blue was a menace. Joan wanted to get rid of her. She thought of writing a murder into the plot, and making this woman the victim. But remembering what I had told her about every character being valuable, she decided to investigate more deeply instead. What was the value of Lady Blue?

She had one of the other characters ask questions of this silent, mysterious character. This questioning revealed that Lady Blue was neither sad nor depressed. She was actually quite content to be sitting motionless, not relating to anyone. Moreover, she believed herself to have a vitally important role in Joan's life. "I am protecting Joan," said Lady Blue, "from the danger of burnout. Whenever she becomes overworked, overtired and stressed out, and won't take a break, I take over. I make her sit in the chair and do nothing. Without me, she might well be dead by now."

The message was obvious. Joan made a decision to incorporate more "time out" into her life, and the Lady Blue part of her agreed to try out a few new activities, like meditation, for example. Smiling as she handed me the script to read, Joan explained that she was no longer at war with this part of herself, but recognized in it a useful ally—one with her best interests at heart.

One aspect of integrity, then, is making sure that we are by now familiar with all the different aspects of ourselves and understanding that they fit together into a whole.

Although the unfolding of the human psyche in the first half of life is well-mapped territory, with markers at frequent intervals, and Erikson and others have attempted to continue the mapping process right into old age,[4] the older we get, the less literature there is and the less we know what to expect. So it is to our inner wisdom we turn, more and more, as each of us proceeds with the integrity project in her own elder years.

Carl Jung spoke eloquently about the change of emphasis at mid-life, i.e. the growing importance of the inner journey as opposed to the outer, and it is to him I have often looked for my best understanding of the basic tasks and challenges of the second half of life and what this integrity thing really means.

According to Jung, the overall goal of the human psyche is to achieve a rounded wholeness.[5] This means acceptance of who we are, warts and all, and an understanding of the value of our so-called shadow, which comprises not only those parts of ourselves we would prefer to disown but also those parts still unknown and unexplored. These are the as yet unlived aspects of our lives; the roads not taken.

This process of re-owning, he called individuation, by which he meant becoming more and more of who we are, and who we can potentially be, right up till the day we die. And dying as our unique, individual selves may well be the crowning point of that process.

Recently, I have enjoyed reading James Hillman's ideas on the subject. In his book, *The Force of Character*, which I quoted in Chapter 16, Hillman states his belief that for each of us, our unique character—that which makes us exactly who we are, like no other—is something to celebrate. He says that as we get older, and that character comes out more and more distinctly, well, that is just the way things ought to be.

And it is not only the "good" bits that Hillman is talking about. Our peevishness and irritability, our impatience and impulsiveness are just as valid a part of our characters as are the virtues for which we are liked and praised. These, also, tend to deepen as we age. And that, too, says Hillman, is perfectly fine.[6]

To me, that is a wonderful, liberating idea. Finally, as we reach old age, we can at last stop trying to fit ourselves into a one-size-fits-all model of the perfect human being and simply start enjoying who we are and where we are, for it is that which makes us truly human—and interesting.

The delight we take in the idea of becoming the sort of old women who wear purple, learn to spit and act outrageously is part of this blossoming of character. Mind you, we must remember that it is only with a lot of preparatory inner work and a deep acceptance of ourselves, just as we are, that we can fully enjoy this aspect of being old. Outrageousness, in the absence of self-acceptance, is merely silly, self-conscious posing. It becomes an immature ego drawing attention to itself, rather than a mature one celebrating its uniqueness.

Now is the time for our eccentricity to come into full bloom. Like an imprint on the world, a tune that lingers long in the air, it is that which will live on after our bodies have departed. It is our characters, rather than our deeds for which we shall be best remembered by those who knew us.

In literature, it is not so much the plots but the well-drawn characters, the folk who are unlike any other, who live on in our culture's memory. Ebenezer Scrooge, Huck Finn, Eliza Doolittle, Jane Eyre—each is a one-off, and it is the unique "isness" of each of them that we recall, above and beyond the tales of their adventures. So it is with us.

Once again, the integrity which comes from full self-acceptance is the vital ingredient here. When we have achieved that inner sense of integrity, feeling comfortable and complete and at peace with our imperfect selves, we express our uniqueness in a natural and unselfconscious way, uncluttered by any need to make an impression or score a point. We are simply who we are. And it is that essence of us which remains when we have departed.

The better we can chart the journey of our lives up till now, the more sense those lives will make to us. Perhaps we shall see them in terms of lessons learned, like a college curriculum, hard at times, and feel as though our death will also be our graduation ceremony into an even higher—and from here, only guessed-at—level of education. Or perhaps what we shall be aiming for is a sense of accomplishment and completion, a sense of tasks well done and loose ends tied off, a roundedness, a feeling of wholeness.

For the elderwoman, then, the life review needs to be more than a mere cataloging of the events of her personal history. Like those puzzle books with the answers in the back, it needs to contain the solutions to some of the questions which have preoccupied her mind over the years.

Why am I here? What is my purpose? What have I come here to accomplish in this lifetime? Am I satisfied that I have accomplished it? What is still left to be done, in the years remaining to me?

At the end of his book *From Age-ing to Sage-ing,* Rabbi Schachter-Shalomi includes a set of eleven exercises, which he calls Exercises for Sages in Training. These are similar to the exercises given to participants in the spiritual eldering workshops which he has been running since 1987. They are based on the concept of life review, and include such items as self-forgiveness, appreciation of the "severe teachers" we have encountered in our lives, and the healing of old hurts. If you are not already familiar with these, I commend them to you as an excellent starting point for the elderwoman process.[7]

Finally, before we leave this topic of looking upstream and seeing the twisting, turning, now fast, now slow river of our lives from the vantage point of today, I would like to suggest to you an optional exercise of my own, which I have used successfully in workshops and with individuals in the past.

EXERCISE
THE TRIPTYCH

For this exercise you will need three pieces of paper the same size. It is an art exercise, but you do not have to have any artistic ability whatsoever in order to complete it. It is an exercise in self-discovery, not a test of talent.

You can use whatever medium you prefer—or a mixture. Crayons, paints, collage (cut and pasted images from magazines, photographs, etc.) are all equally effective.

Picture 1. The maiden

Create a picture of yourself in your maiden aspect. Include all the symbols and images that express who you were as a child and a young woman. What did you look like? What did you feel? What things/people/places/activities/ideas were important to you during those early years? What were your fears? Your triumphs? Your hopes and dreams?

Picture 2. The mother

Now make a picture of yourself as a fully adult woman in the generative stage of your life. Who were you as a mother, a teacher, a mentor of others, a creator, a producer, a maintainer of people and systems? What were your preoccupations? What and who did you love and enjoy/ dislike and fear?

Picture 3. The elderwoman

Next construct a picture of yourself as the elderwoman. What has been lost? What has been gained? What is your harvest? What is your sphere of influence? What is your service to the world? What is the legacy you will leave? How do you look in this, your third age?

When all the pictures are complete, take some sticky tape and on the back, join the three together in a triptych. You might want, at this point, to create a decorative border that both defines and links these three phases of your life into one picture. Then place strips of tape on the front of the seams also.

When you have finished, make folds, so that the two outer ones will fold neatly over the middle one if you need them to. This your triptych.

While the main purpose of this exercise is the doing of it—a kind of life review in visual form—it can also be valuable to show your picture to someone else and explain its symbolism. I have found this a particularly useful exercise to do in groups, with each woman later sharing her triptych and explaining it. Sometimes, the comments and questions of others can provide further insights that we ourselves have missed.

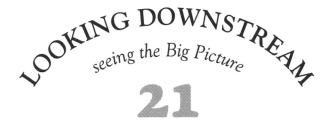

LOOKING DOWNSTREAM
seeing the Big Picture
21

ONE NIGHT, when I was about seven years old, my mother told me what I now call the Parable of the Ant.

Something was bothering me that night, and I was crying. Life felt difficult and confusing. My troubles, whatever they were, loomed mountainously in an overtired mind, and my mother was trying to find words to soothe me into sleep.

"You know," she said thoughtfully, "It's a bit like being an ant, really."

"An ant?"

"Yes. Just imagine that someone had a huge tapestry hanging on their wall. Then imagine you were an ant, and you found yourself trying to crawl up the back of this tapestry. It would be all lumpy and bumpy. The stitches would seem like hills and the dips between the stitches would seem like valleys. There would be little ends sticking out which would seem like fallen trees to you, as an ant. You might note all the different colors of this landscape as you struggled across it, and it would seem to go on for ever and be totally incomprehensible. You wouldn't be able to make any sense of it at all."

As she spoke, I could see the ant, struggling, bewildered, up and down the stitches.

"But if you were you instead of an ant," she continued, "and you were standing in the room, looking up at the tapestry on the wall, you would see what the picture was, wouldn't you?"

"Yes," I agreed.

"So you see with us, it is as though we are ants, struggling with all our problems and feeling confused and bothered, but from where God sits, somehow it all makes perfect sense."

Of all the countless gifts my mother gave me, the gift of that image of the ant on the back of the tapestry was one of the most precious, and also the most useful. It is so easy to get caught up in the details of our own troubles that we lose sight of the Big Picture. Likewise, it is easy to get mentally and emotionally tangled in the problems of others, particularly family members. And it is easy to become despairing or overwhelmed by the problems of the wider world, at every level, from our local community through to the planet as a whole.

When my mother was able to hold up the Big Picture, my confusion eased and I relaxed into a peaceful sleep. Years later, as a psychotherapist, I discovered that a combination of detachment from the details of my clients' problems, a profound compassion, and a commitment to holding within my own heart a sense of the Big Picture was often sufficient to enable people to relax and begin to see a path through their own emotional undergrowth. Sometimes a few words, judiciously placed or an exercise that invited the person into a deeper state of calm were useful adjuncts to this process.

From a Big Picture point of view, every experience, no matter how painful, is a new lesson, and every problem contains a gift within it. Everything is grist to the mill of our growth. Essentially, the simple holding of the Big Picture—the faith that whatever is happening in each moment of our lives is, at some deeper level, exactly right for that moment—is all that we really need to do, either for ourselves or for others. When we are fully committed to that way of being, then what Buddhists call right action flows naturally and easily.

I see the holding of the Big Picture as one of the elderwoman's central functions. At her own personal level, it becomes the pivotal point of her existence as she moves further and further into her third age, dealing with all the issues of aging and the preparation for death. (More about this in Chapter 28).

Within her family or local community, her holding of the Big Picture prevents her being caught up in the swirl of problems and politics and at the same time produces an invisible and invaluable current of healing energy as well as a useful example to follow. At a worldwide level, the same thing applies. A conscious awareness of our spiritual connection with all other life forms is one of the ways we help to heal our planet's ills. Thus even when we are too old to plant trees ourselves, all trees being planted are still drawing sustenance from us.

Compared to the busy involvement of our earlier years, it may seem as though we are doing very little. But ultimately, as I learned from Richard Moss, none of us really has anything to offer except the quality of our presence. And the older we get, the more we realize the truth of that.

Frequently, when we read about the final months and days of terminally ill people, we find observers describing, in awestruck terms, the way in which these people's habitual masks gradually fall away as their bodies approach death, leaving just an immense presence, which seems to fill the whole room in which they lie, opening the hearts of all who visit. There seems no doubt that what we are glimpsing here is the radiance of the soul, coming through ever more strongly as the fabric in which it has clothed itself grows worn and thin. And as Richard says, that is our only true gift, for it is who we truly are. It is our essence. It is our increasing ability to share that essence with those around us which constitutes the most significant service of our elder years. Combined with our increased ability to hold the Big Picture, it makes us extremely valuable for others to have around—and valuable in a whole new way.

During the generative years—those which we have spent in what I refer to as the mothering stage of our lives, giving birth to children or projects or both, actively guiding, teaching, and training others in one way or another—our heads have often been down close to the work. We have been worker ants, busy most of the time. Those were hands-on years. As elderwomen, however, we are moving into the hands-off years. This is the grandmothering stage. We may be equally busy, but busy in a distinctively different and usually more subtle way.

In the previous chapter, we looked upstream, at the journey of our lives to this point. We looked at the influences that others had upon us, and what we made of the raw material that was given us at birth. Each of us took time out to stop and take stock of who she is now. From here, it is time to look downstream. To see where we may be heading and also to see what effects we are having and will—or could—have on the world around us during the last stage of our journey.

By now, if we have had children, they in their turn may be producing children. The students we have supervised are fully qualified and supervising others. Some of those we knew as juniors in our former workplaces have now become bosses. Parents, politicians and police sergeants seem to be getting younger all the time—a sure sign that we are passing into our grandmothering phase.

At this point, we often find ourselves looking critically at those to whom we have passed the baton. Are they doing it right? Have standards slipped?

This is the time to cultivate the Big Picture. Take child-rearing, for example. Let us try to glimpse the Big Picture of human parenting.

A frog lays eggs and goes away. Tadpoles hatch and turn into frogs completely unassisted, according to the ancient blueprint of nature. One day, the frog is fully grown and the instinct to catch flies arises. So, with no teaching except the inner presence of those patterns laid down from all the preceding centuries, the frog goes to find its dinner, find a mate, and continue the life cycle of frogs.

The human baby, on the other hand, emerges still totally dependent upon the care and nurturing of the adults of its species. So the quality of parental child-rearing methods is crucial to its wellbeing.

Whereas the baby frog carries within its genes the historical habits of independent survival, the human baby is programmed for complete dependency. In the psyche of the tiny infant is just one expectation, and that is the expectation of feeling securely held in this new outside world, just as he or she was securely held for those first nine months inside the womb. The newborn even has a grasping reflex, left over from the days when it was necessary to hang on to mother's fur. Gradually, over millions of years, as we have become a hairless species, that instinct has weakened, and the job of holding on has become our responsibility rather than the baby's.

As the weeks and months pass, the baby's instincts for movement, for novelty, for exploration of the world, tasting, sampling and trying out all come into play and he or she leaves the security of home base in the adult's lap for longer and longer periods, pushing the edges of the known world a little farther each time.

Even during those first nine months in the womb, the infant's world was almost certainly not a still and peaceful one. It contained noise, movement and activity. So we can safely assume, I think, that from the very beginning of its existence, an unborn baby's psyche is conditioned to live in a moving, noise-filled world while at the same time being securely held. After birth, the same applies. From the safety of an adult's arms, the baby shares in the business of the world, learns about movement and sound, texture and temperature, light and dark, activity and rest, and all the while that little body—and especially that little brain—are getting used to all these things and preparing for the day when he or she will begin to participate actively in them, rather than being a passive receiver of impressions.

Our distant ancestors intuited these needs, and acted accordingly. However, as they have moved further and further away from their instinctual tribal roots, humans have made many changes in the way they rear their young. Fashions in child-rearing have come and gone over centuries, so there are often radical differences between the orthodoxy of one generation and that of the next. Nevertheless, the ancient patterns still live within our cells. I remember my mother telling me how she agonized over her instinctive longing to hold me when I cried, a longing which clashed directly with the instructions in her parenting book, for in those days, holding babies except to feed them was frowned upon.

In my lifetime, that pendulum has swung. Jean Liedloff who lived with and studied tribal people in the Amazon Basin, far from modern civilization, has discovered that babies reared in accordance with instinctual patterns seemed to grow into amazingly balanced, competent and secure adults. When her work was published, in 1979, it ushered in a whole new era of thinking about child-rearing.[1] Suddenly, babies were being carried in slings down Main Street, just as they are on the paths through the Amazon jungle, rather than being pushed in prams. Babies were sleeping in their parents' beds instead of in cribs, feeding on demand, and feeding at the breast for as many years as they felt inclined. Many of our daughters and sons have been experimenting with these new/old ideas, struggling to stitch them to the rough edges of modern life. This has not been an easy task for them, for it is one thing to follow these precepts in a tribal setting and quite another to translate them into practice in a world of isolated nuclear families, financial pressures, bureaucratic systems and hurtling traffic. Unfortunately, a few of their efforts have resulted in unruly children some of us secretly long to spank.

At the same time, there are many parents who have followed more authoritarian patterns in their child-rearing. They feed, wean and toilet train by schedule, just as their own mothers and grandmothers did. And some of their children are unruly also. What is the right way? It is an ongoing—and important—question.

In education, we see increasing numbers of people turning to the philosophies of Rudolf Steiner, who said that we damage the souls of our children by introducing them too early to the left-brain skills of reading and mathematics and denying them the full time they need to spend in the rich and creative dream world of early childhood. At the same time, the work ethic and left-brain skills are central to the teachings in Montessori-based classrooms. Which is correct? Who knows? There is a lot to think about, a lot of factors to consider. The Big Picture is big indeed.

Joseph Chilton Pearce believes that the three greatest sources of damage done to modern children are over-medicalized birth processes, institutional childcare and TV. His argument about TV is particularly alarming. He points out that not only are children affected by the content of TV programs, but their brain development is actually physically damaged by hours of TV watching. The child, he explains, is born with all its 100 billion neurons already in place, but the developmental task of infancy and toddlerhood is to create a rich network of connections between them. This, the child principally does by hands-on interaction with its world. Passively watching TV creates no connections. However, because of the fast-moving, ever changing nature of TV images, the child's brain is fooled into an expectation of the correct stimulation, so the child keeps watching, rather than moving away out of boredom as it is programmed to do with anything non-stimulating. At around ten, there is an automatic "spring-cleaning" in the brain, which results in physical destruction of any brain cells which have not made connections. Thus the child who has watched hours and hours of TV instead of exploring, and has a poor network of connections, loses brain cells which can never be replenished.[2]

While this knowledge is spreading among certain sections of society, there are still millions who have no awareness of it. I have heard it suggested that such ideas have been deliberately suppressed. Some say the corporate world has a vested interest in the creation of a dumbed down workforce, composed of people of low intelligence but high obedience, which gives no trouble, makes no protest and does what it is told, thereby creating wealth for others.

Even if we do not subscribe to the theory of deliberate dumbing-down, we can see that in the corporate world, too, as in child-rearing, there are many subtle and not so subtle factors and influences at play.

As elders, looking at the whole complex tapestry of modern life, we begin to realize just how many parallel philosophies there are to choose from. There are many different ways to raise a child, to train a student or to run a company, and a wide assortment of belief systems to which we may subscribe.

Equally, there are many different ways to be a grandmother in this society. Those of us who remain involved with grandchildren on a regular basis may find ourselves critical of child-rearing methods that differ markedly from our own. This is a particularly sensitive issue in many families. Some of us judge our children's parenting techniques as too lax; others find fault with what they see as too strict a discipline.

When I first came across the theories of Liedloff and others who advocated the back-to-basics approach, I was highly resistant to them. I remember going to a conference where the speakers were extolling the virtues of the "family bed" and I wrote a scathing report on it for my colleagues who had not attended. It was many years before I realized why I felt so emotional about this issue. It was because it made me feel guilty for not having allowed my children to sleep beside me. What if I had unwittingly damaged them? I confessed those feelings to my daughters, who were now entering their own mothering phase. They held me as I wept, assuring me that no matter what I had or had not done, they had always felt loved and cherished and well parented. I believe that many of the intergenerational conflicts about parenting methods stem from this feeling of guilt. Grandmothers are often loath to consider any new orthodoxy, for to do so is to risk the pain of feeling guilty for "not getting it right." (To them, I say take the risk. Go forward into the pain and out the other side. Your children will almost certainly love you for it.)

After all, who is to say what is ultimately right? Life is forever a work in progress, constantly evolving. Just as in science, or any other branch of human knowledge, each generation, as it goes through the generative phase, builds upon the foundations of the one which preceded it. Sometimes, that involves tearing things down, too.

As elderwomen, whether dealing with family issues, serving on committees, or merely trying to make sense of today's newspaper articles— and to see behind them to the biases and vested interests of those who own the newspapers—we need to be able to stand back and see as much of the picture as we can. We need to see and understand the fluctuation of trends and fashions in child-rearing, education and training of the young and the results these have had on the behavior of the generations they have produced, and to consider carefully what our own opinions on all these matters might be. Above all, it helps if we can tune in to our own inner wisdom and the cellular wisdom we inherited from our ancestors. These are the ancient evolutionary reference books we may find ourselves consulting more and more often. For the elderwoman is freer now than at any other time in her life to ignore the trends, orthodoxies and fashions of her culture and draw her opinions from her own life experiences, from her gut, from her genes and from her heart. From studying both the outer world and the inner world, she has achieved the ability to integrate knowledge and wisdom at the highest possible level

So all of us, in one way or another, during our elderwoman years, can discover that our opinions still count—and count for a lot. The shaping of society is as much our responsibility now as it ever was. It may even be more so. The only difference is in the way that shaping is done. Now, the way we do it is influenced by our tendency to speak from our hearts and guts, our deepening trust in our own wisdom and our efforts not to lose sight of the Big Picture.

Traditionally, it was always the role of the elders to hold that picture, thereby protecting the fabric of their society against any careless damage arising from the impetuousness or inexperience of its younger members. In our own times, this safeguard has become almost lost. As Robert Bly has pointed out, we are fast becoming a "sibling society" where youth rules, age is discounted, and information is prized more highly than wisdom.[3] Reversing this trend is our task. It is a daunting one, but fully achievable.

However, we do not have to achieve it single handed. Our numbers are growing fast. And whatever we do, however small and seemingly insignificant, is still important. The arts and skills of deep vision are applicable everywhere and at every level of our lives. Neither my grandmother nor my mother had large egos. Both were shy and modest women. Yet their influence, in its own way, was mighty.

At my mother's funeral, as I stood to speak my eulogy to the huge assembled crowd, I could think of no more fitting tribute to her than to tell them about the Parable of the Ant, a simple story, with a great teaching in it. From there, it may go on to touch a thousand hearts and make a difference in ten thousand lives. Who knows? Yet she would never have suspected, in her lifetime, that her words to me at that long-ago bedtime had achieved anything at all, except perhaps to help me calm down and go to sleep so that she could go back to doing her crossword puzzle.

As her grandchildren, in their turn, stood beside her coffin and spoke of her influence on their lives, I realized that they valued her teachings in just the same way as I had valued those of her mother, the grandmother I have spoken of so much in this book. And there was a similarity, too, in the type of things they named. Like me, they spoke of simple, enduring values and how they hoped to incorporate these in a form that fit their own lives. This, to me, was yet another validation of my claim that while the footprint left by each elderwoman who walks on the Earth is different, the footprint of an elderwoman has a recognizable shape—and of how important all our footprints are in the great scheme of things.

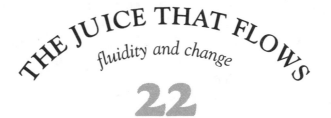

THE JUICE THAT FLOWS
fluidity and change
22

A MALE DOCTOR once commiserated with me about my misfortune in having been born female. I stared at him in amazement. "But I *love* being a woman," I said.

"Oh really?" He seemed surprised. "Most of my women patients don't."

I found that strange. To me, there is a special, wonderful juiciness about living in a woman's body, a juiciness which seems to connect us deeply to the earth, to the sap of trees, to the ocean tides which wax and wane, as we do, with the moon.

Of course, we don't start off juicy. The body of a little girl is small and light. Buoyant. Dry and compact, like a tightly folded bud.

With puberty comes that first wet heaviness. Breasts swell. We begin to bleed. This is a huge change, bringing with it an inner turbulence as our bodies learn to accommodate to the hormones of womanhood and to prepare for the possibility of growing babies. Babies, who are aquatic creatures for all of their intra-uterine existence, re-enact that ancient drama of evolution which began in the sea, and need us to be liquid.

It seems that an increasing number of women, these days, experience problems with fertility and may not be physically able, for one reason or another, to conceive a child, even though they desperately desire to become mothers. For such women, the juice of their bodies may seem to mock them, as every month's bleed renews the anguish they feel—an anguish too deep for comforting. For we are all inescapably juicy for all

197

those years, and we cannot dry out—except by surgical removal of our ovaries—until the calendar dictates it. And since we are multi-dimensional beings, our juiciness operates at an energy level, as well as a physical one. All of us—whether biological mothers or not—nurture the world with our juice in a million, million ways.

A friend of mine, who occupied a senior position in an organization, suffered the ruination of her career when she chose not to return to work fulltime after the birth of her child. She had asked for her position to be redesigned as a job-share situation, and she and her colleagues had worked out exactly how this could be done—to the advantage of everyone. But the answer was no. So this woman's unique and juicy energy, which had done so much to enhance and transform the organization in which she worked, could flow there no more.

Electricians refer to the energy in the wires as "juice." The huge capacity we have, during that whole section of our lives between young adulthood and menopause, for productivity in one form or another, is also a sign of our juiciness, our ability to keep the work wheels turning by means of physical and mental energy, enthusiasm, strength and stamina.

Unfortunately, when we let our energy juices flow in the work world, the demand on them is often greater than we can manage to sustain. For the juice of female energy does not come in as steady a stream as the juice of men. It fluctuates more widely than theirs. It has rhythms—some of them predictable, some not. Times of high activity, times of rest. Times of inward contemplation and times of outward action. Women are cyclic. We bleed. We gestate. We give birth. We suckle infants. We caretake. We cry. We have hormonal headaches and hot flashes, and the occasional day of lassitude in between days of high output. The workplace, however, is a notoriously alien and unfriendly environment which takes little account of nature. Our biological reality is seen—if it is seen at all—as an inconvenience. Most of society's institutions are tailored to fit men and machines, rather than women and children. So although many women have succeeded, over the last fifty years, in gaining their rightful place in the work world alongside their male companions, they have usually been forced to repress and ignore the needs of their own female bodies and psyches in order to do so. It has been a high price to pay. They have seen little alternative but to override their natural female rhythms (and often to short-change their children) in order to fit into a male-ordered world.

Menstruation, pregnancy, childbirth, lactation and menopause have all taken second place to this need to keep the alpha males happy and the steady-state machines running. Unable to redesign the work and the workplace, they have tried to redesign themselves.

I believe it is time to call a halt to this sort of sacrifice.

So when I hear talk about the return of the Goddess, the emergence of a New Age of gentleness and light and feminine energy, I like to remind people of the very practical, ordinary, down-to-earth things that every one of us can do to bring back respect for the feminine. For any change will be mere window dressing unless it affects the fundamental structures of our society. If we truly respect and value the feminine, then we need to insist that our institutions be adapted to the biological realities of women—not the other way around. Flexible hours, telecommuting, decentralization, baby friendly workplaces, job-sharing—there are many, creative ways to do this. The exploration has barely begun.

Just as solar power can efficiently run appliances despite the alternation of sun and shade, so could society's machinery adapt itself to the fluctuating juice of its female workforce if it wanted to. It is up to us to work together to make this happen.

Sure, there have been some gains since the first suffragette chained herself to a railing. At least on paper, women have achieved equal rights and equal pay and a vote—for what it is worth. We have maternity leave, and a few have flexible work hours—all these are a good start. But we still have a long way to go. And in times of high unemployment, when people are scrambling for jobs—not to mention the trend towards using cheaper offshore labor—the gains we have already made can be lost overnight. The elderwoman, who has been right through the cycles of wetness and dryness and understands the female rhythms better than anyone, can certainly make her voice heard in this debate. If enough of us do so, the needed changes will occur faster.

Changes need to occur not only in our own society but also for the women in other countries whose conditions lag far behind our own—such as the exploited women of the *maquiladoras*[1] who work grueling hours for minimal pay and for whom pregnancy often means instant dismissal. Maternity leave, for them, is but a distant dream. We need to speak out on their behalf as well. All our voices count, and our actions count even more. If every woman in America and Europe chose fair-traded, non-sweatshop products for her every purchase, sweatshops would probably be gone within a couple of years. That's how powerful we are.

Unlikely to happen, you may think. But who knows what miracles may result from the actions of this rising tide of elderwomen which is gathering now? In the U.S. alone, the number of post-menopausal women will soon reach fifty million. If even half of these become true elderwomen, plowing back into society the wisdom they have gained, think what an influence that could have on the whole course of history!

In order for that to happen, however, we have to learn to combine the passion of our beliefs with the compassion of age. Our voices need to be firm, authoritative—yet gentle. For as Theodore Roszak suggests,

> *As we lay the foundations of a postindustrial moral order, it is essential for elders to assume a greater role in our affairs. That role ought not to be a mere extension of midlife getting and spending. Far more challenging is the task of remaining involved and responsible, but in a new key, one that sounds a note of gentleness and ethical responsibility.*[2]

As I see it, for women to be able to play a full part in this revolution, we must first of all be comfortable with the process of change. Rather than walling ourselves off in safe enclaves, we need to stay aware of the ways in which the wider society is moving. Yet we also need to protect ourselves from its excesses—its noise, its hype, its restlessness—and free ourselves from its constant pressures, particularly its pressures to get and to spend. It is a delicate balancing act, involvement and detachment combined. And each of us has to work out the ways in which that balance may be accomplished in her own situation. There are no general recipes.

One of the chief ways in which the forces of consumerism hook us is by tapping into our fears of becoming old—particularly our fears of *looking* old. The fading petals issue is, for many of us, our Achilles heel. So the very same inner work that allows us to move smoothly into elderhood is also our best guarantee of effectiveness as elderwomen. If we accept the process of change, accept aging as simply another of these great changes which we, as women, are used to going through, then our sales resistance will be automatic. We shall be beyond the reach of temptation.

It seems like an irony. That which made us feel the most womanly—our juiciness, our fullness, our raw energy, our sexual attractiveness—is the very thing we have to be able to give up graciously in order to be complete as women. It is the woman who no longer tries to be what she once was, but fully embraces what she now is, who is the most womanly of all. The elderwoman is more completely a woman than any other female person, for she has lived each stage of the cycle.

Not only are there women who have difficulty negotiating the change from mother to crone; some have difficulty with the earlier move from maiden to mother. Many women, like the patients of my long-ago doctor, curse their femaleness because it feels like a handicap, a brake on their ambitions. They dislike their own wetness, their own heaviness, their very connection to the Earth which bore them. They dislike their rounded bodies and yearn for the hard, the thin, the angular. They want to remain maidens forever.

Our Western culture has fostered this image, particularly in the prolonged love affair which marketers and advertisers have had with extreme youth over recent decades. Think of the waif-like models whose barely-teen-plus-sex images in advertising border on pedophilia. By reflecting young people back to themselves in an ever deepening narcissistic back and forth movement, until fantasy blurs with reality, the marketing/Madison Avenue axis has created, among other things, an epidemic of anorexia.

I have known many casualties of this war on biology—like Jane, the young woman who once told me she felt burdened by her wetness. She longed to be light and dry, to fly like a bird. One day, trying out the idea of fasting as a spiritual exercise, she had discovered that after two or three days of not eating, she felt wonderfully light, almost euphoric. It was as though she were weightless. Like the mythical story of Icarus, she fell in love with lightness and with the idea of flying. With the lightness, eventually came dryness, as she ceased menstruating. But this type of lightness becomes an addiction, and like many other addictions is potentially fatal. Icarus flew too close to the sun, and when his wax wings melted in the heat, he crashed to his death in the sea. This young woman came close to meeting the same fate. But she survived.

Three years later, after conquering her addiction, she became pregnant. I saw her again shortly after the birth of her child. Her body had filled out.

Her breasts were huge and full of milk. She was still bleeding slightly, from the birth.

As she greeted me, I exclaimed how well she looked. She smiled. "I feel so *heavy*," she said. "And so *wet*! I'm dripping from everywhere!" We laughed together. "How does it feel?" I asked her, remembering her love affair with lightness and how difficult it had once been for her to bear even the fullness of her stomach after a meal.

"Absolutely wonderful," she replied.

Just as there are maidens reluctant to move into motherhood, there are also mothers propelled into physical cronehood before their psyches are ready for the challenge. One woman who, before cancer came into her life, was robust, sexy and strong, with three young children still in her care, wrote a poem about how she felt after chemotherapy:

> *Vitality fled hand in hand with sister Fertility*
> *And only the hairless crone remained, loose bellybag*
>   *wrinkles and empty titdangles*
> *Picking over the tattered threads of her youth*
> *Searching for meaning.*[3]

Not an easy place to be in for a woman barely forty.

So being female brings a whole sequence of changes and challenges, to be met either with fear and apprehension or with courage and acceptance. And for some of us, when the sequence is somehow disturbed, the challenges are even greater.

Here, then, is yet another map of our development—a uniquely female one. From the dry lightness of childhood, we pass through the doorway of puberty into the wetness of womanhood, and into four decades of activity in the world. For many of us, this will include the amazing bodily changes of pregnancy, birth and lactation. At menopause, there may be a struggle as our body juices dry up and we experience the rigors of estrogen withdrawal. But then, finally, as the juice of our womanly lives transforms into wisdom and compassion, we attain the free, sweet lightness of old age.

I don't know about you, but I am enjoying the journey. That is, when I don't spoil it for myself by being afraid of change. Fear of change seems to be the main thing that makes most people miserable. Acceptance of change—the nineteenth in our list of elderwoman principles—is perhaps the hardest of all to incorporate into our own, personal lives, since it must inevitably include acceptance of our own dying.

simplicity • deep vision • passion • compassion • non-attachment • Earth-centeredness • comfort • connectedness • respect • creativity • delight • lightness • enoughness • heart-listening • peace and quiet • authenticity • responsibility • radical aliveness • acceptance of change •

Intellectually, we know that life is eternal flow. But in our frantic need for security, we often try and dam the river, obstruct and deny the reality of change. We fear the current, fear letting go into the flow of life.

For me, facing each change in one's life is like diving into deep water. If we fall off the cliffs of change fearfully, terrified of drowning, and we struggle and splash, believing that we shall sink—we inevitably do. But if we dive trustingly, believing that the water will hold us up, it does so and we float effortlessly.

By the time we reach elderhood, we should by now have amassed enough experience to teach us that this principle invariably holds, and have learned to trust it in everything we do.

If, during this last third of our lives, we can fully embrace the inevitability of flow and change, and risk entrusting ourselves to the deep water of each new, unknown moment, we can position ourselves to face the last great challenge—the challenge of death—with equanimity and acceptance. This life's learning will thus reach a full and satisfying completion and our end will be our graduation.

Well, it sounds good. The truth is, though, that when it comes to change, the unknown, and especially death, I am as scared and diffident as everybody else I know.

A male friend of mine, who as a child had been too terrified to jump from the high diving board, carried the shame of that for over twenty years. Then, on a cycling trip around New Zealand, he had the opportunity to bungee jump. Trembling with fear, he stood once more on the edge, but this time, as he stood there trembling, high above a deep gorge, with the river far below, it was a vastly bigger and deeper drop which now lay before him. His own history flashed into memory, the swimming pool, the fear, and the ignominy of climbing back down the ladder. This time, though, there was no going back.

"I didn't have a choice," he said. "They counted down—five… four… three… two… one… and the roar of their voices filled my ears. It carried me. I shut my eyes and took that step…"

He came back a changed man. For him, the bungee jump was a transformational experience.

Men need to make their own opportunities for meeting change, for the pubertal change from boy to man is the only one pre-orchestrated for them. For women, particularly if we give birth and suckle children, living in these bodies provides many such opportunities. So we get more practice than they do. We are lucky.

I still like being a woman, very much. But I hope that even after all this practice, at the end when I need some help with letting go, those voices will be there for me, carrying me, as I face the inevitability of that last scary step, out of this woman's once-juicy body—five, four, three, two, one… and off the edge.

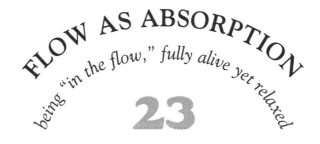

FLOW AS ABSORPTION

being "in the flow," fully alive yet relaxed

23

MY GRANDMOTHER invariably hummed as she went about her daily tasks. She hummed as she cooked; she hummed as she sewed; she hummed as she did the laundry. There was a calm, unhurried quality in the way she did everything. I cannot recall ever seeing her in a flap. I loved to listen to her humming. It seemed like such a happy sound.

It was a quiet, fairly continuous humming, usually not of any recognizable tune. What was recognizable, however, was a certain quality it had, unlike any other sound I knew. Even to think of it now flips my memory back to my childhood, to the delicious smells of Grandma's kitchen and the visual memory of her busy hands. Hands which could rub fat into flour until it resembled fine, soft breadcrumbs, or deftly twist and pinch the edges of a bulging Cornish pasty. Hands which guided the hot iron, as it nosed its way into the corners of a shirtsleeve, conquering every crease. And above all, hands which could do a miracle I never learned to emulate, and that was to place a straight and even running thread along four or five inches of fabric with one rapid little wriggle of the fingers ("just a dressmaker's trick," she said).

When my first child was about four years old, I began to notice exactly that same quality of humming in her solitary play. It almost always arose when she was doing something creative, whether it was drawing a picture or building with her blocks or Lego. I came to know the message of that little hum. It meant she was deeply absorbed and very content.

It was years before I realized that I, too, hum. I caught myself at it one day, as I was walking along the street, lost in reverie. As I stopped at a traffic light, suddenly I noticed myself making this gentle inner sound.

I love to live simply, as my grandmother did. But I am also a creature of my times. I love to bake bread in my old wood oven, but I also love to surf the Internet while the dough is rising. I suffer, as so many of us seem to nowadays, from never having enough time to do all the things I want to do. Instead of the slow, unhurried pace with which my grandmother went about her daily tasks, I always seem to be dashing from one thing to another, glancing at the time, fretting at the lateness of the hour. Even in so-called retirement, the habits of a busy lifetime are slow to be relinquished. Though there is no longer any need to watch the clock, grab a hasty meal or hurry to finish a letter before the mail goes, I still find myself doing all of those things, many times in a week, chasing satisfaction in all directions, like a hyperactive greyhound, rather than slowing down and entering fully into each experience so that satisfaction could then find *me*, instead.

So the moments which are most precious in my life these days are those times when I, too, find myself quietly humming. Those are the times when I really know that I have succeeded in finding just the right pace at which to do something, just the right something to do, and just the right way of doing it.

Psychologist Mihalyi Czikszentmihalyi from the University of Chicago has made a study of what he calls the phenomenon of Flow.[1] Flow is what happens when we become fully absorbed in an activity, when mind, heart and action all point in the same direction. It can happen in sport, in music, in kneading dough, in digging, in rock-climbing, in sex—or virtually anywhere. The only prerequisite for this gentle, wonderful state, this special suspended time-out-of-time, is that we are relaxed yet fully attentive, totally absorbed in whatever we are doing. Not only are we optimally contented in these times of flow, we are also at our most efficient, creative and effective, no matter what the activity. Any sportsperson will attest to that; it is the moment when he or she suddenly and wonderfully hits form.

It is my contention that the simple life, like the life of my grandmother, lends itself to the achievement of this Flow state. And according to Czikszentmihalyi's research, Flow enhances our overall wellbeing and sense of satisfaction with life.

The life of most elderwomen is ideally suited to the achievement of Flow. Unless we are still holding down paid jobs, we have the freedom to organize our own time in a way that suits us. So if we still find ourselves— as I quite often do—in that old familiar harried state, where there no longer seems to be enough time for all the things we want to do, then we need to stand back and take a good look at ourselves.

What we may discover is that underneath all our dashing about is a fantasy. It is a fantasy which says "One day, I'll stop living like this, but, of course, right now I can't because..." (You fill in the gap.) The fact is, of course, that unless we make the effort of will to rearrange our thinking, our habits will not change until our bodies finally force the issue, either slowly by the loss of strength and stamina or suddenly by illness.

People who have faced a medical crisis often tell us that their way of thinking was forcibly changed by the experience. Theodore Roszak says that when he faced his own medical emergency he recalled a quip he had often heard—but never till that moment truly taken seriously—which is that nobody on his death bed ever regretted that he had not spent more time at the office. Suddenly it dawned on him that there was nothing on his list of things to do which could not, if necessary, be seen to by somebody else.[2] We are all capable of stepping off the treadmill, if we really want to. Believing that we can is the hardest part.

For me, this has been one of the hardest elderwoman tasks to accomplish—this voluntary shift into my grandmother's gear. I am still struggling with it. And I know this is so for many others. Perhaps it is because we have no clear cut moment that defines our movement into elderhood. A few of us may have had the ceremony of retirement, complete with gold watch. But many others have drifted out of the workforce rather than jumped. And no one has given us classes in new ways of structuring our days. So even in retirement we tend to follow the old habits, which are to keep taking on new activities until we suddenly reach saturation point.

As in hasty eating, the signal usually comes a little too late for comfort. It tells us we are *too* full rather than almost full. And then we have the problem of working out what we have to give up in order to return to the comfort zone.

There is a better way. That is to measure the amount of time we spend in quiet, relaxed mode. I call it the humming test. If I go for a whole day without humming—I know I am too busy.

The ancient Greeks had two words for time—*chronos* and *kairos*. Chronos time is the ordinary everyday time, measured by our clocks and wristwatches. Kairos time has a different quality altogether. Kairos time is what we find ourselves dropping into when all our senses are absorbed in an activity, whether we are painting a picture or making love or stopping to watch, in fascination, the bird which has just flown down to take breadcrumbs from the windowsill. In other words, kairos time is what we experience when we achieve that Flow state.

Children, who are all born into kairos time, have great difficulty adapting to the chronos-obsessed world of their parents. "Hurry up, you'll be late for school" comes as a rude intrusion into their world . I remember once watching a group of schoolchildren painting and trimming a large papier-mâché model they had made. There was no chattering—just a quiet absorption in the task. The atmosphere in the room was peaceful and pleasant. Suddenly, the shrill ringing of the school bell crashed into the quiet, shattering the mood. I watched the grimaces, the looks of disappointment. I watched the reluctance with which they tore themselves away. I saw chronos break up their morning into adult-driven chunks. And I felt sad. How much better it would be, I thought to myself, if they could have stayed there until the task was complete. How much better if our school programs were flexible enough to follow the contours of the activities themselves, rather than breaking up the day into arbitrary sections. States of Flow would be encouraged. Tasks could be completed and the satisfaction of completing them could be fully felt.

I know it can work that way, too. My mother, who was a grade school teacher, for many years ran a tiny one-room school in a small English village. She did away with strict timekeeping and let each child work and develop at his or her own pace. Nature's own scripting, which starts every normal child off as a curious, exploring being with a massive appetite for learning, was allowed to continue expressing itself, rather than being destroyed by rules, regulations and schedules. In nearly twenty years, she never experienced one single case of dyslexia, learning difficulty, hyperactivity, attention deficit disorder or unruly behavior in that classroom. To me, that speaks volumes for the importance of letting our children maintain their natural affinity with kairos time as much as we possibly can. If we did, the adults they grow into may not be the stressed-out workers who collapse in front of TV every night. And when the time comes to retire, they may have fewer difficulties in making the necessary adjustment to elderhood.

The elderwoman phase of our lives is the one in which we finally have the opportunity to return to that freewheeling blend of kairos and chronos that my mother's pupils enjoyed. We need to welcome and embrace that opportunity.

We should all, I think, spend as much time as we can in the state of Flow. We can all do with more humming in our lives.

Then, not only shall we be at our most contented, but, like the sportsperson hitting form, we shall be at our most creative and efficient, too. If our primary task, as elderwomen, is the use of our harvested wisdom to nurture the world around us, then our efficiency in doing it must surely be a good thing. So let's hum as often as we can.

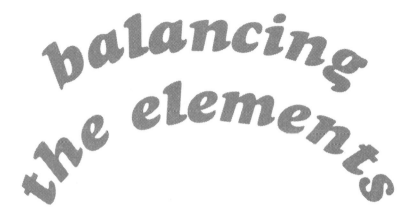

balancing the elements

HONORING BOTH MOTHER AND FATHER

remembering the real rules of nature

24

THE MOST important thing about the elements is, of course, the way they interact. For the world to work properly, they all need to be in balance. So now that we have concluded our tour through some of the earthy, airy, fiery and watery aspects of our lives, I want to devote the remaining chapters to this concept of balance. Balance, as you may already have guessed, is another important item on our list of principles.

• simplicity • deep vision • passion • compassion • non-attachment •
•Earth-centeredness • comfort • connectedness • respect • creativity •
• delight • lightness • enoughness • heart-listening • peace and quiet •
• authenticity • responsibility • radical aliveness • acceptance of change •
• balance •

Let's begin by looking at a serious imbalance which is behind a lot of the problems our world has been experiencing. I call it the mother/father imbalance.

Most of us have childhood memories of male authority. This may have been personified by our own fathers or other family figures, or perhaps by teachers or clergymen. Beyond those were two figures of even greater male authority. One was the somewhat stout gentleman in a red suit who lived at the North Pole and delivered toys to us at Christmas, provided that we had complied with the house rules for most of the preceding year. He delivered these gifts overnight, bringing them right into our homes, like some super-conscientious UPS driver, via the chimney. (The houses we lived in when I was a child always had open fireplaces and chimneys wide enough to be credible, but I have not thought to inquire whether modern parents in centrally heated houses and apartments have found creative ways to amend the story. I guess they must have.)

In addition to him, we were taught that the CEO of this whole enterprise we call the Universe is another elderly gentleman, who wears a white robe rather than a red suit and lives in a place called Heaven. The exact location of Heaven is never given, but is referred to as being somewhere in the sky. Wherever it is, we are also destined to go there eventually—again provided that we have kept to the rules—but not until we die.

Both these elderly gentlemen love us and reward us for good behavior. Both keep tabs on us too, so that if we do not perform to the standards expected, you can bet your life they will know about it. And both may be contacted. Santa prefers to be approached through the mail, except during December when certain privileged persons also get to sit on his lap and speak to him directly about their hopes and desires. God, on the other hand, has a wonderful free voicemail system called prayer, so you can leave messages any time, from anywhere. (The assumption that he listens to his messages is called faith.)

So who personifies mother?

In some form or another, we all experienced a mother figure. She may have been—if we were lucky—one consistent person, and our own birth mother. Or there may also have been an adoptive or foster mother, a grandmother, or someone else who took care of us, day to day. It was our mother figure who explained the rules, policed the rules, provided nourishment, shelter, solace. She was the one who kissed us better when we fell. She was angry when we displeased her. Maybe she told us stories. In all her many ways, she taught us, moment by moment, hour by hour, week by week all the basic things we needed to know to take our place in the world as human beings.

Often we are not even consciously aware of what she has taught us. But she created us out of her body, fed us from her body, sheltered us in her arms, supported us in her lap, and in every moment of that creating, that feeding, that sheltering, that supporting, she taught us lessons. From her we absorbed, through our skins and our bones, our mouths and ears and eyes, knowledge of how the world is—knowledge of good and evil, of pleasure and pain, of how people live in the world, what language and communication are, and how it feels to be human and alive. A mother can be both loving and angry. She is gentle and sometimes scary. She is everything. She is the matrix within which we have our being. The words "matrix" and "mother" have the same root meaning. She created us, and she has the power to destroy us also. Like any other baby creature, each of us knew this instinctively.

If I asked you, out of the blue, "What rules did you learn when you were a kid?" your mind might flash back to grade school. You might think about times tables or how it was forbidden to throw spit balls. But the most important lessons of all, the really basic lessons that form the foundations of who we are, as human beings, and how we take our place in the world, we learn way before school, and the earlier we learn them, the more deeply they are part of us—and the less aware we are of them. Things we learned before we had language are often invisible to us, since we have no words to express them, but we carry them in all the cells of our bodies.

Robert Fulghum's clever essay, *All I Really Need to Know I Learned in Kindergarten*[1] rang true as soon as I heard it, for I knew that some of the most basic and important learning we all do in our lives is that learning that happens in the very early part, when we are so very open and flexible and trusting. Then, our horizons are limited to our little neighborhood, or before that, to our mother's arms, or the inside of her womb. She creates our world. And the inner map we make of that world is the map we carry out into the wider world. We navigate from that map—with some notes scribbled on it from later, of course—for the rest of our days.

It is interesting, that we are more likely to be consciously aware of the Ten Commandments or the Highway Code than we are of the basic rules of living as an animal in the world of plants and animals and other living things—rules like "Eat Only What You Need" or "Kill Other Creatures

Only to Eat" or "All Species are Equally Essential to the Web of Life" or "It is OK to Get Sick and Get Old and Die."

It appears that the Rules of the Father—those codified ones we learn at school, at church, at Scouts etc.—are the visible rules: things like Talion Law (An Eye for an Eye and a Tooth for a Tooth) or My Country Right or Wrong. The Rules of the Mother—all those foundational ones we have learned from conception onwards—are the invisible ones. Like the fact that our mother has the power to destroy us and that we must, therefore, conform to the shape in which she molds us. If we don't, we won't get fed and nurtured and loved. And that one that we learned while still in the womb, which was that if something is not good for her then it is not good for us either. Anything that poisons her, poisons us. (That is a key one.)

You can see where I am going with this, can't you? Whatever is true at an individual level is also true at a universal level. As babies, we learned the basic rules of life, like which was up and which was down, and how to eat and how to love, directly from the bodies and beings of our mothers. And as animals, humans originally learned the basic rules of being a living creature on the Earth from Mother Earth herself. From watching her, observing her, feeling her in our bodies, we, as a species, learned about up and down, day and night, moon and stars, seasons and cycles, and about procreation, life and death.

I don't know about Santa Claus, but certainly God was not always thought of as male. This seems to me a really interesting correlation: in the days when God was thought of as a universal mother rather than a universal father—and we now know from our studies of history and archeology that this is how it was for probably twenty thousand years, up until about 2,000 B.C.—the pace of change was slow and organic.

Round about the same time that agriculture began, the idea of God as Father began to emerge. After that, within the space of a few centuries, everything speeded up. What we now know as "modern civilization" began to evolve. It was a runaway process.

By the nineteenth century, we had placed so much emphasis on the Rules of the Father that we had almost totally forgotten the Rules of the Mother. By the twentieth century we had become so clever—learning to fly higher than birds, creating machines that had the power of a thousand horses or could do sums faster than any person who ever lived, changing the course of rivers and shifting entire mountains—that we thought we were invincible. We could do anything, understand anything, control anything.

What we forgot was that despite our clever brains, we are still animals. As animals we are still part of the web of life. And we are still bound by the universal Rules of the Mother. The penalty for breaking those rules is destruction. So we have come to the edge of our own destruction.

It has been an interesting and exciting ride. It is great that we now have jumbo jets and the World Wide Web and electric wheelchairs and all the other amazing inventions of the creative human mind. But it is not good that the lungs of the world—the rainforests—now have emphysema because we have damaged them so terribly. It is not good that the equivalent of several jumbo jets full of mothers watch a beloved child starve to death every day because the resources of the world are unfairly distributed and because those who have more than their share (which is most of us in the West) won't let go of anything. It is not good that the continents and oceans are polluted and species are going extinct at the rate of dozens a day.

It is all very depressing to talk about and even to think about. But it is important to understand the issues so that we can see what each of us can do to help restore the yin/yang balance.

Single parent families manage all right, usually. But they do so because every single parent knows deeply in his or her heart that ideally, every child really needs two parents. He or she therefore works really hard, either to provide two different kinds of parenting, or to bring in other friends or family members or community people to plug the gaps.

I believe that elderwomen are crucially important in the task of bringing the Mother and Father rules into equal balance, importance and respect. One of our chief tasks is to think hard and try to remember what all the Rules of the Mother are, so that people can start listening to them and obeying them. Only then will life on Earth begin to thrive again.

Our aim should not be to establish the superiority of women over men. It should not be to throw out the Rules of the Father in order to bring back the Rules of the Mother. It should be to honor and value these two equal but different qualities which are in everything. Whether we call these qualities male and female, yang and yin, or something else altogether, our aim should be to value them equally, to respect and enjoy their difference, and to integrate them.

At an individual level, by spending more time and effort being quiet and actually listening to our own bodies we can learn to become increasingly aware of what they are telling us, of how they are asking us to treat them. This is listening for the Rules of the Mother as they are to be heard right within our own physical bodies. We are literally made from the molecules of our mother's bodies. And we are all made from the molecules of our Earth. So we are all part of the natural living Earth. Therefore the voice of the Mother echoes within this very body in which you walk and sit and live. You do not even have to go out into the woods to commune with nature. You *are* nature. So for a start, you have only to listen to your own true insides. It is all in there.

At a relationship level, we have to stop this silly squabbling about who is superior and once and for all really get it that male and female are equal and different and complementary. The oriental yin/yang symbol expresses this complementarity perfectly. Each completes the other, each contains a bit of the other, they fit perfectly together, and they are equal in size and beauty.

Finally, on a societal level, we have to rescue the Rules of the Mother from the dark ages they have been in, and start making them conscious. We have to start honoring and respecting and living them, side by side with the Rules of the Father. And if they clash—which sometimes they do—then sit down to talk about it. From that dialogue, we shall grow in understanding. A child grows and thrives when parents can sit down at the table together in mutual respect and resolve their differences with creativity and with dignity.

Just imagine how it might be if Mother and Santa Claus were to sit down at the kitchen table some time in early December and discuss the differences in the rules. Santa's rule is, of course, that if you have been good you get lots of toys. Mother's rule says that the more toys you have, the more you want and that for every toy you get, resources have to come out of the ground. She has another rule that says the way to feel good is to share loving, connected feelings with other people, and that that is more valuable than toys. So maybe they would come to a compromise that says you can still enjoy Christmas, and Santa will still bring stuff, but what he might bring are things like a coupon that entitles you to a massage or to some guitar lessons—or some home-baked cookies with your initial on. And Santa might agree to have all the presents wrapped in special "Christmas squares"—squares of pretty fabric saved from year to year for re-use, and tied with satin ribbons—so nothing gets wasted and no more trees have to die for the sake of making a surprise.

To me, the whole concept of caring for trees is a wonderful illustration of the vast variety of ways in which the elderwoman's message may be delivered. Whether we spend our summers in a volunteer team, restoring ancient forests; chain ourselves to a redwood in defiance of the loggers; carry a cloth bag to the store so that we can say no to a paper sack; create a picture or poem about trees; or simply talk to a tree and listen to its reply, (see the exercise at the end of this chapter) really doesn't matter. What matters is that our actions, no matter how simple or insignificant they may appear, are part of the great project of restoring balance to the Earth and bringing the Rules of the Mother into greater awareness. Even one more tiny spark of awareness, in the mind of just one more person, is precious.

Every time we make a point of listening to what the Rules of the Mother have to say, we see new ways to make our ecological footprints lighter.

The older I get, the more I realize the importance of this hidden set of rules and the importance of bringing them out into the open—articulating them, discussing them, making them conscious. I am convinced that this is the natural task for the new generation of elderwomen, a task which may be accomplished in such a wide range of ways that there is a way to fit every single one of us.

My grandmother knew nothing of this. Not consciously anyway. But many of the Mother's rules were a part of her, and some of them she even spoke. Her gems of folk wisdom came out in the form of timeworn sayings. Some were trite little injunctions like "Waste not—want not." Who has not heard this a thousand times? And yet how many of us really think deeply into what it means? When we make a personal decision not to continue subscribing to the consumer ethos which has come to rule the society we live in, and begin to follow, instead, a private ethic of minimizing waste in our lives, whether it be a waste of our own energy on meaningless pursuits, a waste of our talents by not being courageous enough to try something new, a waste of our time vacuously watching TV or a waste of valuable resources like oil, wood or coal, we start to become more and more aware of the bounty which is all around us. When we become fully aware of that bounty, we shall want for nothing—ever.

Once this sense of soul-richness has developed in us, there is absolutely nothing we need to do to persuade anyone to follow our example. Simply to let ourselves glow with it is advertisement enough.

In the summer of 1996, on my third visit to Kripalu, I was introduced to a wonderful exercise which I have since made into a regular practice. This was the exercise of listening to a tree. You may like to try it. The results can be surprising.

We spoke in Chapter 7 about the notion of learning respectfully from other creatures. Here, we apply the same attitude to trees. I have included this exercise here because I believe that trees are deeply in touch with the Rules of the Mother and excel at reminding us what those rules are.

EXERCISE
LISTENING TO A TREE

If the weather is not too cold and wet, and there is no poison ivy, it is great to do this exercise in bare feet, if you can. There is something about being barefooted outside in the garden or in the woods which makes us more aware, more careful, more humble. Without shoes, we cannot so easily trample things. It is we who will get damaged if we do not step carefully. So the playing field upon which we meet the rest of nature is suddenly more level than if we were to walk in boots. But if you cannot do the exercise barefoot, keep your shoes on. It is still a great exercise, even in gumboots.

All you need is a tree. Any tree. Each species of tree seems to have a different energy, all its own, and to speak in a particular voice. My favourite tree is the oak. I love the ways oaks talk.

Find your tree and approach it reverently.

Make touch contact in some way, either by placing your hands on its bark or leaning against it or both. You can close your eyes or leave them open, whichever feels most comfortable and natural.

Let yourself relax, and take as much time as you need to clear your mind of extraneous thoughts. Come into a gentle, meditative space.

Be aware of all the sounds, not in a naming or interpreting way, just in a pure awareness of sound—the sort of awareness you would bring to a symphony concert. Imagine that you ARE at a symphony concert, and simply listen to the symphony of sound which is in the air around you.

As you do this, you will become more and more aware of all the sounds that are happening. You may be surprised how many layers of sound there are, at this moment, layers you had not even noticed before. Allow yourself to become exquisitely aware of them all.

When your sense of sound has sharpened, switch your attention to the senses of feeling and smell and sharpen them in the same way.

Feel the texture of the tree. Explore its surface with your hands. Smell it. Smell the air around you and feel its touch on your face.

Now, with your mind clear and empty, and your senses sharpened, begin to listen deeply for the voice of the tree. It will probably speak in whole sentences, directly into your mind. Or it may guide your senses to a particular sound or sight or sensation that seems to carry a strong message. If you wish, ask it a question. Not a yes/no question, but an open question, like "Do you have any advice for me today?"

You could ask the tree to tell you more about the particular Rules of the Mother, by which it lives its life. And, if you love trees, and want to do the best you can for them, ask how you can help. Listen to the answer, in whatever form it comes to you.

When you feel, intuitively, that you have learned what you needed to learn from the tree, speak some parting words and release contact.

Please remember, before you leave, to thank the tree for whatever it has given you.

It is traditional to leave a gift in exchange. I often take a hair from my head and wind that around a twig or tuck it into a crevice in the bark. My gifts seem to me paltry, compared to what I gain from this exercise. But trees are great givers and this never seems to bother them. They are invariably delighted that someone bothers to stop and listen to what they have to say.

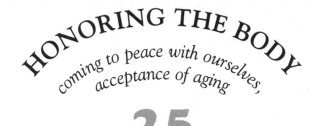

HONORING THE BODY
coming to peace with ourselves, acceptance of aging

25

I WANDERED one day into one of those New Age stores, a bookshop cum health food store cum natural health center, replete with dolphin pictures and rainbow decals.

The air was sweet with aromatic oils, and the gentle, tinkling strains of ambient music soothed the ear. It seemed like a pleasant antidote to the rush and bustle outside. I made some purchases, and as I was leaving, picked up a flyer for a women's health forum.

The first sentence that caught my eye was "Beat the menopause without HRT."

Beat the menopause?

Why such warlike language? I wondered. Why should we want to *beat* something which is so much a natural and inevitable part of every woman's experience?

It reminded me, yet again, that as women in this culture, we have been conned into declaring war on our own bodies without even realizing what we are doing.

Some fifteen years ago, researching for my work on menopause, I interviewed many dozens of women about their attitudes to menstruation in general and menopause in particular and found that a great many of them experienced their natural female rhythms as a nuisance at best and at worst a downright curse, reflecting that for many, that expression "the curse" seemed a literal truth. This made me sad.

For a long time, my focus was on articulating a different view of menopause. I wanted other women to see menopause as I did—as a rite of passage, an opportunity, and a doorway to personal development and spiritual transformation.

Gradually, over the years since I wrote *Transformation through Menopause*, that focus has widened. Now I can hear myself speaking not just about menopause, but about the tragedy of a society in which people—particularly women, but men also—are at war with the very bodies in which they live. It is like walking out into the garage, picking up crowbars or machetes and attacking our automobiles, splintering the paint, smashing the windows, slashing the tires—and then wondering why those cars will no longer carry us so comfortably to the places we want to visit.

We seem to have split our minds off from our bodies to an alarming degree, both as individuals and as a society. This has been particularly destructive for women, whose cyclic, rhythmical patterns are at variance with the mechanical, steady-state structures of the workplace, and who have therefore, as I mentioned in Chapter 22, had to deny so much of their essential nature in order to win political equality with men. And it has denied us the joy and the natural acceptance of the aging process. So in this section of the book where we look at our relationship with our physical bodies, the first thing that comes to mind is this tragic split and what we can do, as elderwomen, to heal it. For only if we heal it completely in ourselves can we be of any use in the greater healing that is needed—the healing of the split between human beings and the body of the planet.

When we split off from our bodies, from the natural cycles of sleeping and waking, of energy and rest, of eating and digesting, and try to impose our will on them in the service of some "higher" need, like making money or pleasing an employer or meeting a deadline, then it is a kind of violence we do to ourselves. You never see a cat deprive itself of sleep in order to finish an assignment.

The only reason we can do it is that we have reserves for those times when extra effort is imperative. I expect a lioness with cubs to feed would stay out hunting a while longer, even if she were sleepy, rather than come home empty-mouthed and let the family down. Or if she herself were being hunted, she would stay awake long past her bedtime if necessary, to ensure her own safety or the safety of those she loved.

It does not hurt us occasionally to postpone lunch or miss a few hours of sleep or run extra hard to catch a train, for our bodies are designed by evolution to hold enough in reserve to meet such demands from time to time. We have a complex and beautifully designed stress-coping mechanism which enables those reserves to be quickly accessed and later to be replenished. Both lions and people—in fact, most animals—are designed that way and it seems to be a good design, for it has served us all for millions of years. The problem comes, however, when we dip into our reserves continually and they go down and down without being replenished.

Then, like a car with broken shock absorbers, we can no longer cope with stress. We have burned out. Many animals, if stressed beyond their ability to replenish, will simply die. We do too, but more slowly, insidiously, without noticing.

"Increasing energy levels for women of the twenty-first century" promised the flyer. A benign promise, surely? But I read the small print.

"The twenty-first century woman has changed a lot with added responsibilities, business and careers… If you are finding that today's fast pace is leaving you exhausted then come along and find the secret of how to increase energy levels."

Ah. Never mind that today's fast pace is killing more and more people with heart disease and other stress-related conditions. Never mind that today's fast pace is creating more psychosis, neurosis, suicide and depression than ever before. Increase your energy levels and all will be well.

Wait a minute, I thought. Let's look at this another way. Perhaps the increasing incidence of fatigue, especially in women who are trying to keep up with today's fast pace is a kind of warning sign. Like the canaries the old-time miners used to take down into the mines to warn them of toxic fumes, maybe these women are showing us a danger we need to heed.

Sure, we need ways of coping with fatigue, and it is nice to have increased energy levels. But let us not do it without thinking long and hard about how we shall use that extra energy. Let's not be conned into simply increasing our energy levels—whether with amphetamines or benign herbal substances or even yoga and meditation—and then not looking at the Bigger Picture. Let's not just use that extra energy to run faster and faster on the treadmill. Rather let's look critically at the treadmill and do something, in our own way, in our own lives, towards stepping off it, and lets encourage others to do the same.

Each small action taken by the individual is the beginning of a pond ripple. Just one frog plopping into the lake, and the ripple begins, and widens, touching places which that individual frog may never know nor comprehend, washing against farther shores than he or she has ever reached.

Perhaps it is better to say no to the promotion that would bring more money but would take up more hours, more energy, more time away from the kids and then to compensate by, for example, giving away or selling something that is expensive to maintain. As anyone who has downshifted to a simpler lifestyle will agree, there are many beneficial side effects to that process apart from saving money.

An old friend of mine from Australia gave up his high salaried job in an advertising agency and went to work instead for a charity organization, doing fundraising. Adjusting to a much lower pay scale, he sold his luxury car and bought a little Mini Moke instead. He not only had some extra money to spend, but the car was more economical and, best of all, he discovered a whole new world. Bowling along with the top down, he found a subculture of the open road. Suddenly, he could make eye contact and smile. Now he felt more at one with cyclists and pedestrians than with other drivers—except those with open vehicles. There was a certain camaraderie, he found, a banding together of "real" people who chatted at traffic lights, united by their exposure to the open air and sky and the feeling of freedom that comes from being out in the fresh air while everyone else is sealed in the insulated capsule of a car. He liked it. Driving became a constant source of amusement and surprise.

One of the bibles of downshifters—people who voluntarily simplify their lives—is a book entitled *Your Money or Your Life*.[1] And the literal truth of that title lies in the fact that in the mainstream of our culture people are giving up the full enjoyment of their lives in order to make as much money as they can, not realizing what a poor bargain they may actually be getting.

So yes, let the women go to this forum and learn how to increase their energy levels. That will be wonderful. But I do hope that they also take some time to look at why their energy levels need increasing. Is it that they are already dipping daily into their reserves, trying to run faster and faster on the treadmill of consumer society?

I have long been a proponent of natural health. To me, however, that does not merely mean using herbs instead of drugs. It is not just about finding less toxic substances with which to medicate our bodies; it is about healing that very split which made them succumb to disease in the first place.

The underlying philosophy of natural health is based on an honoring of the natural processes of the body, co-operating with them and learning from them, rather than trying to outwit or "beat" them.

I know very well, from many years of working in the health field, that—unfortunately—most of the medical profession is still firmly entrenched in the extremely masculine magic bullet/warfare model of fighting disease, the legacy of several centuries of mechanistic thinking.

What is called for today, therefore, is a feminine/co-operative/ transformational model supporting health, a model that sees symptom as message, crisis as opportunity, and illness as a sign that something is wrong with the way we are living our lives, individually and/or collectively.[2]

I still run women's groups, and I know that inside many a woman who is trying to keep up with today's fast pace is a rebellious little whisper which suggests that maybe those low energy levels are a sign that the real problem is with today's fast pace, and not with her. That whisper needs to become a shout. A shout first within her own body, her own life, and then a shout out loud. A declaration that she will no longer be conned into living her life—and dying her death—according to this sick society's crazy agenda.

Every woman listening to her inner whisper, every woman making a small change in her life because of that whisper, living in closer allegiance to her own body and its rhythms, is a hero. She will make ripples, whether she tries to or not, whether she even knows it or not.

It bothers me when "alternative" practitioners ape the medical model; that model which says, "if it hurts, fix it quickly, for discomfort of any kind is a no-no;" that model which talks about "fighting" and "beating." When this language is used by so-called alternative practitioners, in my opinion, they are not being alternative at all. All that is happening is a substitution of herbs and oils and essences for drugs. It is a step in the right direction, to be sure, for natural substances are generally preferable to synthetic ones.

But the underlying philosophy is the same. There is no real shift in the things which make us sick in the first place.

I believe that when we are truly in touch with our bodies, our discomforts have much to teach us. I am certainly in favor of natural remedies, but I fear that in our rush to find a quick-fix, we can so easily miss the deeper message. Our discomforts are for feeling into, exploring, learning from. They are invitations. If we have learned to think like this, then the discomforts and aggravations of an aging body will make us neither indignant nor scared. Instead, we shall explore them with interest and compassion and listen to the signals they are giving us.

Unable to resist, I telephoned the young male herbalist who was running the seminar, challenging him on his choice of wording and the images it invoked. I suspected that he had not really thought deeply about it and was unconsciously using "medical model" language. He told me that he agreed with my philosophy and explained that he had merely worded his flyer in a way that he thought would attract women who were looking for alternatives to HRT. He had not thought about the deeper implications.

If he did manage to incorporate these into his seminar, then I hope his participants came away from the session determined to *explore and fully live* their menopause process rather than to "beat" it. I hope that any career-minded, stressed out woman who came looking for increased energy levels went away not only with new ways to increase her energy levels but also with new ideas as to why those energy levels were so depleted. Maybe she was determined to continue trying to be Superwoman and kill herself in the process. If that is what she consciously wanted, then fair enough. But I hope that he was able to lend support to that subversive whisper inside her that told her maybe "today's fast pace" is a con game. If she can honor her whisper, it may become a roar.

The big task that faces us is to begin rearranging societal structures to suit human rhythms, both male and female, rather than suppressing, ignoring or subduing those rhythms—particularly the female ones—in order to conform to a system based on the mindless, soulless hammering of the consumerist economic machine. Learning to honor our own biology is the first step in learning to honor that greater biology of the mighty being called Earth, of whose body we are but cells.

It is a huge task. Too big to tackle, you might think? No, I do not believe that it is.

Since we are talking now about balance, it is important to look at all the ways in which the elements of our physical, bodily lives may be balanced in order to function in the best way possible throughout the remainder of our days.

The first step, I believe, is to honor these bodies in which we walk around—to see them as the miracle they are—and to make a vow, here and now, that we will, from this moment forward, do our best to respect them and never, if we can possibly help it, make war on them in any way or even think of them with anything less than love and acceptance, no matter how ancient and decrepit they may become.

If we have this mindset, then many of the things we do and say will automatically be influenced by it. We shall be ambassadors for change without even trying. We do not need to create opportunities to campaign for a new attitude to the body and its messages, for the opportunities will always present themselves. A word here or there, a few sentences in a letter to a friend, something we may say to a neighbor, or even to a stranger we meet on the bus might be catalysts for a change in the way that others think about their bodies too.

I remember once, long ago, reading a snippet in a magazine about an elderly man who went to ask a doctor's opinion about pain in his knee. When the doctor tried to dismiss him with "Oh, don't worry about it, it is just something that happens in old age," the man retorted, "Well, in that case, why don't I have a pain in my other knee? They are both the same age, after all. So please attend to my knee."

That exchange stuck in my mind for probably forty years. Until then, I had never thought much about the physical process of aging, nor about how old people are routinely discounted in our society, nor about what a savvy elder might say in response to such dismissive behavior. That silly, tiny—and probably apocryphal—story encapsulated all three. The insight it gave me remained, like a seed lodged in my mind, growing into something quite significant in my later life. And in just the same way, something you or I might say can lodge in the mind and memory of another. Though the chances are we shall not know whether or when it does so, for the transmission of wisdom is often as invisible as the transmission of a virus—and as unpredictable.

As a therapist and a workshop leader, I have often re-encountered people who tell me: "There was something you said years ago that I have never forgotten." Then they repeat what it was. Not only do I almost never remember having said it, but if ever I did, it was a throwaway line. Usually, they were words mistakenly attributed to me. Conversely, on those occasions when I have uttered what I thought was something incredibly wise or significant, no one ever remembers hearing it. So I am convinced that there is absolutely no point in trying to look or sound wise. There is only one thing to do, and that is to be authentic. The rest is serendipity.

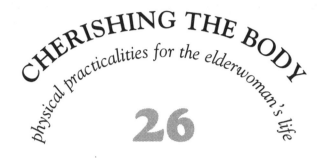

CHERISHING THE BODY
physical practicalities for the elderwoman's life

26

WHEN YOU have lived in the same house for fifty years, you know every crack and creak of the floorboards. You can walk around in the dark without bumping into anything. Your fingers find their own way to the light switch, turn the faucet to just the right spot, understand the catches on the cupboard doors. The walls you have painted, the pictures you have hung, all speak to you in a language of familiarity. So living for half a century in the same body should, one assumes, have created just such a deep knowing in us. We should by now know all there is to know about the moods and preferences of our stomachs, the limitations of our limbs, the degree of pressure we can safely put upon our lungs and hearts. By this time we should know how to respect our individual livers, care for our particular pair of kidneys and lavish attention on our personal envelope of skin. If we don't, then it is certainly high time we learned.

Just as houses need more care and attention as they age, so do bodies. So in this chapter, let's look at some of the ways in which these aging bodies need to be cherished.

Here is our list of the principles which turn an old woman into an elderwoman. How might these relate to the cherishing of our bodies?

• simplicity • deep vision • passion • compassion • non-attachment •
• Earth-centeredness • comfort • connectedness • respect • creativity •
• delight • lightness • enoughness • heart-listening • peace and quiet •
• authenticity • responsibility • radical aliveness • acceptance of change •
• balance •

Well, in clothing, for example, maybe our need to follow fashion fads has given way to a delight in pleasing ourselves (comfort/non-attachment). For many of us there is a sense of relief in paring our wardrobes (simplicity/lightness) down to a set of well-made, well-matched garments, the colors and textures of which add to our sense of wellbeing, conform to our personal aesthetic and comply with our need to avoid anything which, in its manufacture, has harmed or exploited anyone or anything (Earth-centeredness/responsibility).

Released at last from the dress codes of the corporate world, and no longer having an image we need to uphold—or at least, not anyone else's—we now have the freedom to experiment, if we care to, with types of clothing we have never tried before (acceptance of change). I like watching the way my favourite elderwomen handle this issue. They are all delightfully different. Liz is famous for her bright, rainbow-colored clothes and her crazy, incredible hats (radical aliveness). Jenny wears sweat pants and sneakers almost everywhere and rarely dresses up at all (comfort); while Mary, who had never given much thought to clothes, discovered some years ago that she had been wearing the "wrong" colors for most of her life, whereupon she threw out everything and started again. We can indulge in the fun of dressing up if we feel like it (creativity/delight), while feeling free from any pressure to do so; we can say to hell with convention and wear whatever we like, whenever we like (authenticity). So each of us is different. What we may have in common is that the older we get, the more likely we are to be aware of the environmental and social issues around clothing (deep vision/passion/compassion).

As with clothing, so with food. Since each of us is biochemically unique, it is much more important to recognize our own individual dietary needs than to follow some prescribed regimen. Just as a mother soon becomes expert in discerning the meaning of her baby's different cries, by now we should all have fine-tuned our responsiveness to our own body's signals so that we, rather than anyone else, are the greatest experts on them. We should have learned, by this stage in our lives, how to interpret their various messages and know better than any nutritionist what to feed them and when (heart-listening/respect).

However, if we have been too busy up till now to think about all this, it is time to do some intensive study of ourselves and our inner workings. Not only do we need to gain a general sense of nutritional principles, but our own dietary needs are likely to depend on our particular body type. There are various typologies which attempt to explain and classify the natural groups into which humans physically fall, and if you have never looked at any of these, I recommend you do so, for they are excellent tools for self-understanding. You may well find that many of the foods recommended for your particular type—whether based on ancient wisdom, such as the Ayurvedic teachings of India,[1] or the yin/yang scale of macrobiotics[2] (balance), or on something modern, such as the recently developed blood type system[3]—are the very ones to which you have been intuitively drawn.

Once again, enjoyment, love, (food cooked lovingly seems to nourish far more than any other kind), aesthetics, simplicity and comfort are all important, as well as the nutritional value of our food. So are matters like seasonality, the yin/yang balance, our own particular allergies and sensitivities, and the environmental aspects of food production and distribution. Learning to discriminate between the body's genuine call for a certain food and signals of addiction to non-nutritious items, for example the craving for sugar, alcohol or coffee, demands a high degree of awareness and discernment. All these matters deserve study, for we owe it to ourselves to cherish these bodies by putting into them only what will do them good, what will nourish, strengthen and fortify them and delight them without incurring a health penalty.

At this time in our lives, there may be a change not only in what we eat but also in the way that we eat it. If we have spent years gobbling down hasty meals so that we can go shopping in our lunch hour, reading a book instead of focusing on what we are eating, or snacking instead of preparing proper leisurely meals, now is the time to slow down and savor what we put in our mouths (peace and quiet). Now there is time to chew slowly and derive maximum pleasure from the taste and texture, just the way we did with the raisin meditation in Chapter 9. Food becomes less like filling up at a gas station and more like enjoying a concert (enoughness/delight).

Whereas the spacing, content, location and duration of our meals may previously have been determined by outside forces, many of us will have more freedom now in terms of what, when, where, how and how often we eat. If we have partners, they, too, may welcome the opportunity to be more flexible and to tailor a routine more suited to their own body's needs (compassion). My own partner and I have developed a style and pattern of eating which takes account of our very different rhythms and yet preserves the pleasure we get from eating a sit-down meal together at least once a day (connectedness). We also take turns at cooking that shared meal, which builds even more freedom and flexibility into our days. I love it when it is his turn to cook and I can work on in the garden till dusk and sit down to a meal he has lovingly prepared.

My friend Parvati takes so many vitamin and mineral supplements that she practically rattles when she walks. Parvati is a sucker for health magazines and catalogs. She has a cupboard stacked with little bottles, though by now she has forgotten the reason why she takes half the things in it. Daphne, on the other hand, maintains that no one who is eating a clean, healthy diet, rich in organic vegetables, wholegrain cereals, beans, nuts, fruit and sea vegetables should need any supplementation at all. Daphne, as you may have gathered, is a purist in lots of ways. Though to give Daphne her due, she does have a diet exactly like that, and at sixty-five is as fit and strong as a racehorse. But most of us ordinary mortals have a slightly less than perfect diet. So a bit of supplementation here and there seems like a good idea.

In recent years, there has been a lot of scaremongering about osteoporosis in older women, and many people have been panicked into taking hormone replacements (HRT) in an effort to protect themselves against what they fear is a dangerous but inevitable loss in bone density. The savvy elderwoman, knowing how important it always is to look at the Bigger Picture (deep vision) and heed the wisdom of her inner skeptic, is aware that this is at least partially driven by the drug companies' search for a lucrative market. Certainly, there are some women with a family history of osteoporosis who are at risk and may therefore benefit from HRT. Also at greater risk than average are women who have undergone premature or surgical menopause or women with a history of anorexia or amenorrhea. But for the rest of us it is not likely to be a problem unless we smoke, take steroid medications, drink a lot of alcohol, coffee or cola drinks, eat a diet bereft of minerals and vitamins, and/or lead a very sedentary life.

It is true that for about five years right after the periods stop, the bones apparently refuse calcium, and their density decreases. However, they start absorbing calcium once again when this five to seven year transition stage is over. Eating plenty of calcium-rich plants (such as leafy greens) combined with regular weight-bearing exercise is the best way of building and maintaining healthy, flexible bones and protecting ourselves against osteoporosis. Cooked greens provide abundant, highly usable calcium. One cup of cooked broccoli, plantain, turnip or mustard greens contains about 200 mg calcium. One cup of cooked collards, wild onions, lamb's quarter, or amaranth greens contains about 400 mg. Cider vinegar, taken with these, ensures good absorption. Common calcium-rich herbs such as nettle, sage, chickweed, red clover, comfrey leaf, raspberry leaf, borage, dandelion and horsetail can also be useful, either in the form of herbal infusions or made into a tincture by soaking the fresh leaves (plus some clean, crushed eggshells) for about six weeks in cider vinegar. (One cup of infusion or one tablespoon herbal vinegar equals 250–300 mg calcium) Other calcium-rich things to add to one's diet are tahini, tofu, oats, seaweed, sardines, salmon and yogurt. A low-protein, low-fat diet rich in complex carbohydrates (whole grains) is best, from a calcium point of view, since foods high in protein but low in calcium (such as red meat) result in calcium being excreted in the urine.[4]

As well as eating a healthy, sugar-free diet and adding herbal infusions and tinctures, many people (myself included) take calcium supplements, just to be sure. But it is important to ensure that these are in an easily absorbable form, such as calcium-fortified orange juice or chewable tablets of calcium citrate. (Beware of synthetic sweeteners in the cheaper brands.) All calcium should be taken with Vitamin D and magnesium, and most proprietary brands include these. Spending time with one's skin exposed to the sun also produces Vitamin D, of course, although with some of the ozone protection now missing from our atmosphere, due to pollution, it is wise to cover up during the middle part of the day as a protection against skin cancer.

If you are taking hormone replacements, it is still not clear whether you have to go on doing so for life in order to prevent fractures. It is possible that women who stop HRT and who are several years past menopause may trigger a loss of bone density at that point.

While on the subject of HRT, I might add that an increasing number of women, disillusioned with its promises, are abandoning it. Though some women claim that they feel good on it, many stop taking it after a short time, disliking the side effects.

We should all be aware, too, of the abuse of animals which is involved in the production of at least one popular brand. This substance, one of the top five most prescribed drugs in the United States today, is made from pregnant mare's urine. It contains at least twenty horse estrogens none of which are native to the human female body. In order to produce the drug, more than seventy-five thousand pregnant mares, on farms in the U.S.A. and Canada, are kept tethered in stalls for seven to eight months of their pregnancy, with specially designed pouches strapped to their bodies to catch their urine. Water is restricted, as that would dilute the hormones. Exercise is denied, and when the mares give birth, they are immediately re-impregnated. The thought of animals suffering this way, just so that women can avoid the discomfort of hot flashes, fills me with horror and rage. Especially when I know, from my own experience, and the experience of many other women like myself who embraced menopause as a natural stage in our lives, that hot flashes and other menopausal symptoms can not only be alleviated by natural, herbal and dietary means, but can also be used to great advantage for our own personal growth. Once I saw that I was being transformed by my own menopausal process, each hot flash assumed enormous symbolic importance. Like birth contractions, these dynamic, dramatic signals from my body filled me with awe and excitement. I would not have missed them for the world. (I love it that today's women call them "power surges.")

If, for whatever reason, you embark on HRT, I hope that you insist on researching carefully the brands which you are offered and refuse any which contain equine estrogens. Be aware that several brands of HRT contain hidden tranquilizers of one sort or another. At least one contains chlordiazepoxide (Librium). So read the small print!

If anyone on HRT wants to wean herself off it, I recommend the technique of shaving a little bit off each day's dose, over a long period of time, so that the body does not notice what is happening. It always amazes me how few people use this straightforward, practical method of reducing any medication they no longer wish to take. Tablets can have tiny pieces taken off with a sharp knife, capsules can be slid open and rejoined so that some of the powder can be shaken out, or, if they are all of a piece, they can either have a tiny end snipped off or be cut open and the contents decanted into empty capsules which can be obtained from a pharmacy. I have used all these methods, and they all work.

The other key factor in supplementation for older people is antioxidants. Controversy still rages about what actually causes aging, but most theorists seem to agree that free radicals circulating through our bodies in increasing numbers as we age can cause ill health and accelerate the aging process. Vitamins C and E, selenium, grape seed, Co-enzyme Q10 and gingko biloba have all been recommended as useful supplements for older people, and new contenders for "wonder herb" and "wonder supplement" appear regularly. So unless we are to finish up like Parvati, with extensive—and expensive—collections of pills, we may need to maintain some healthy skepticism. My solution is to ring the changes. I have two or three of the recommended items on hand at any one time, but take only one of them each day. I am not sure how useful this is, but it certainly cannot do me any harm. And at such low doses, it does no harm to my pocketbook either.

Let's look now at exercise. As you know, there are three types of exercise: aerobic, which tones the heart and lungs; stretching, which keeps the joints and muscles flexible; and muscle-building. All three are important to us throughout our lives and never more so than in old age. Muscle-building exercise protects against osteoporosis, aerobic exercise keeps our hearts and lungs healthy—thereby making us less prone to a whole range of degenerative diseases—and stretching exercises keep us supple and less at risk of falling or injuring ourselves by sudden movement. An orthopedic specialist told me once that more people injure themselves getting out of bed than they do on the sports field. Like everything else in our lives, this is something it pays to do with full attention rather than with our minds hurrying ahead of us to somewhere we think may be more exciting.

Women who exercise regularly live an average of six years longer than sedentary women. Brisk walking is probably the best all-round exercise there is, and all of us should aim to walk a few miles a day, if we can.

There are so many possibilities to choose from that every one of us should be able to find enjoyable forms of exercise. And enjoyment is a key factor. If you hate the water, don't swim, even though you know it might do you good.

If, as old age advances, we find our mobility restricted, whether by disease, accident or loss of strength and stamina, we shall need to adapt our exercise regimens accordingly. It is a challenge to be more and more creative. You do not need to go to a gym to lift weights. A house brick, a two-pound bag of flour, a parcel of books, can all do duty as gym equipment. Those simple strips of thin rubber that physiotherapists use cost a dollar or two and can be used in umpteen different ways to exercise a host of different muscles. You can exercise in bed, in the bath, in a chair—anywhere. If your legs no longer work, you can still dance with your arms, your hands, your fingers.

If we are to be able to adapt continually as we age, without a sense of failure or loss, then it is important *right now* to accept the probability that our strength and mobility will be reduced, if not sooner, then later. As Sherwin Nuland has pointed out in his no-nonsense, factual book about the dying process,[5] no one dies of old age any more. Every death certificate names one disease process or another as the cause of death. When the curtain comes down, there are just a few common ways for it to fall. Whether the heart packs up before the kidneys fail or the liver ceases its function before the lungs stop breathing does not really matter a whole lot. All those things will happen at the end, anyway. And knowing that should not give us a sense of failure. Dying is no more a failure than is being born. If we have no expectations about how long we should live, how fit we should be, how much or what kind of exercise—or, for that matter, about anything else—we should be able to do as we get older and replace all such expectations with an attitude of interest, openness, fascination and general expectancy, we shall be true elderwomen. That is the secret of how we take radical aliveness right through into our final moments. We say yes to everything: to failing strength, to flagging energy, to loss of balance, to failing eyesight, to disease, if necessary, and to death itself. Just as we would cherish a loved one who is terminally ill, we cherish these bodies of ours until the last.

This brings us to the last important aspect of body-cherishing, and that is our wishes as to how this body should be treated once our soul has left it.

If we have made simplicity a hallmark or our later lives, it would be nice to think that this same simplicity would feature in our dying and in the return of our bodies to the Earth.

With this in mind, I recently bought a book which answered every one of my questions on the subject.[6] From it I learned that I could, if I wished, write out a "living will" to ensure that my life shall not be artificially prolonged on life support. I can ask that my coffin be made of recycled and biodegradable material, such as cardboard, and that if I decide to be buried rather than cremated, which would seem to me to be less polluting, I can be placed beneath an oak tree in a newly-created woodland, as part of a re-afforestation project.

Making all these decisions now will release my loved ones from having to second guess me at a time when they need to be dealing with their grief and concentrating on creating their own rituals for letting me go.

Unfortunately, while the general information in this book is wonderful (it even includes designs and full instructions for DIY coffins) many of the resources which it lists apply only to the UK, where the book was published. Right now, as I write this, there are fewer such resources in the U.S., but the movement towards simplifying, naturalizing and re-owning death—just like the natural childbirth movement which has been re-empowering birthing women since the 1960s—is gathering momentum. Lisa Carlson's excellent book *Caring For Your Own Dead* is a good place to start. For as Lisa says,

> *Almost everything the funeral industry sells interferes with our natural return to the earth, and few know what that involves. By understanding what happens to the body after death and demystifying funeral options, our end-of-life decisions prior to death may be less fearful to face.[7]*

Her book includes a number of U.S. resources, including a state-by-state listing of laws pertaining to death and funerals.

Still very much alive (and working hard for the cause she believes in), Lisa decided to write a letter to her children, explaining her thoughts and ideas on the subject of her own funeral.[8] I was very touched by her sentiments, as they sound so much like my own, especially when she laughs at the image of herself as *a plain, ordinary, not-very-good-looking, wrinkled, not-in-great-shape-and-therefore-baggy-in-places mom—a mom who got into more mischief than most, with many embarrassments for all of you, I'm sorry to say.*

She remarks how funny it would be to find herself, a self-styled "outrageous older woman" finishing up, at the hands of the funeral industry, perfectly posed in a casket full of satin and crepe.

So I would like to close this chapter with her words on how she would like her body to receive its final act of cherishing:

I'll tell you what I really want—it's very easy: "Ashes to ashes and dust to dust." I want a plain pine box. No, not plywood with all the glue and formaldehyde. I want a plain wooden box, one that will return naturally to the soil, as I'd like to do.

"Plant" me under an apple tree, or—better yet—a flower garden… It feels strangely warm to "see" myself becoming one with the earth, to picture my elements feeding new life. That's the way I want to go—that's the way I want to come back again—as nourishment for a beckoning flower.

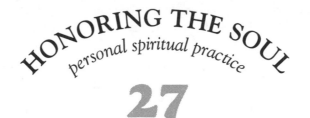

HONORING THE SOUL

personal spiritual practice

27

WAITING IN line at the airport check-in counter, I have company, and plenty of things to watch and to think about. It is only later, with my boarding pass in my pocket, alone in the ladies washroom, that I suddenly become aware of the fear in the pit of my stomach. It is always there, lurking in the shadows of my mind, whenever I fly.

Walking down the jetway, stepping across that threshold, into the stomach of the great silver bird that will lift me thirty-five thousand feet and whisk me across continents, is a definitive moment. Now there's no turning back. I'm committed to the journey. When those doors close, my life is entirely in someone else's hands. That's a scary thought.

Then, after the taxiing, comes the moment of take-off. Faster, faster, then suddenly the nose points skyward and we roar up into the clouds. The surge of power pushes me against my seat. And the strangest thing happens. My whole being becomes filled with the exhilaration of that wonderful moment. Fear falls away. And for a little while, until the screen of my mind becomes cluttered once again with the trivia of existence, I experience the sensation of absolute, total trust.

It seems surprising that after sixty-plus years on this planet, a lifetime of reading inspirational books, attending personal growth workshops, meeting enlightened teachers and having many thousands of experiences which have validated all those teachings, it can still take a ride in a Boeing 747 to remind me of how it feels to trust the pilot.

I think the reason it works is that once we are on board a plane, we are simply forced to have that trust. There is no other choice.

In ordinary life, however, our clever little egos have so many ways of tricking us into believing that they, rather than our souls, are in charge, and so many ways of distracting us, that we spend most of our lives believing ourselves to be in conscious control of everything and totally forgetting that there is actually an immortal soul in the cockpit.

When things go wrong, or appear out of control, or when we start experiencing large or rapid changes in our lives, we tend to cling, white-knuckled, to our seats, whimpering in fear. And yet, if things get bad enough, eventually we give up. Paradoxically, that act of giving up, if it really is a deep giving up of the attempt to control and a true surrender to the inevitability of the moment, can sometimes lead to a breakthrough in spiritual growth.

This is not the "Oh dammit I give up" of the petulant ego, or the listless giving up that comes with depression. It is a response to inevitability which releases a burst of energy, since all the energy previously tied up in avoidance, distraction and denial is now suddenly available for use.

The truth is, of course, that we can always trust the soul to pilot our craft wisely and to know, like a migrating swallow, the true direction of our journey, even if that direction is one the ego might not like or approve. After all, only soul has the proper map. The map we carry around in the pockets of our everyday minds is but a blurred photocopy of one tiny section, so how could we possibly presume to navigate from that? It would be as though Jules Verne's hero, Phineas Fogg, had taken a page from his local street directory and tried to find his way around the world with it.

The huge plane burrows upwards through the clouds and suddenly we are out in the clear blue spaces above, bathed in eternal, unchanging sunlight. Those clouds below suddenly appear small and unimportant, just like my fears. How strange it seems, now, that I could ever think there are days when the sun literally stops shining. Because, of course, it never really does, it 's just that some days we lose sight of it because of the cloud cover. And I close my eyes and smile. I think to myself, "I must remember this. Whenever I have doubts I must simply recall this moment. And I must remember that I can always trust the pilot."

But I'll forget, of course. I always do.

For much of my life, I held the naïve belief that there were a few truly enlightened people who were able to remain permanently in that open, trusting space. I used to believe that when I, too, became "truly enlightened" then I would be like them. So I spent a lot of time trying out various spiritual practices, in the hope that one of these practices, or a combination of them, would eventually lead me to this enviable state of enlightenment.

I was at least wise enough to know that although every now and then one reads or hears of some person who became enlightened by a kind of random act of grace—a blessing that came from nowhere, unannounced— most of the people who have this experience had already prepared the ground with some kind of spiritual practice. For, as Richard Moss always says, enlightenment is an accident—but practice makes you accident prone.

Gradually it dawned on me that fully enlightened folks are pretty thin on the ground. To be sure, there are gurus aplenty, men and women whose whole beings seem suffused with an intense energy that has the power to inspire and grace others by their very presence. They are people who have attained a very advanced type of consciousness. Many have achieved powers that we call paranormal. Nevertheless, they are still human beings. And usually, in their private, behind-the-scenes lives, they are as subject to whims and difficulties and bad hair days as the rest of us.

This need not detract from their value to us as inspirational figures. For the deeper teaching they are offering us is, in fact, that enlightenment is not the destination. It is the journey itself.

This reminds me of a weekend yoga workshop I went to once, many years ago.

The leader was a charismatic young man with deep, dark eyes and a voice like honey. He always seemed very mystical, and yet very calm and present. It was as though he were in touch with a source of energy that the rest of us mortals could only dream about. People flocked to him and he had a large group of disciples who hung on his every word.

I never did become his disciple. For one thing, I had known him, in all his ordinariness, since he was a university student, and I could not quite fit him into the role of spiritual guide and guru, even though my friend Parvati worships the ground he walks on. Also, I am too much of a rebel to be anyone's disciple. But I have attended his workshops and meditation groups from time to time, and he has given me many subtle gifts over the years.

The workshop I remember so well was the one where he asked us to assume the *ekapadasana*, (the tree pose where you stand on one leg with the other foot resting against your thigh). I had done this *asana* before, but with my hands in front of me, in prayer position. This time, he instructed us to raise our hands, still with palms together in the prayer position, above our heads, and leave them there, "Until something happens."

He did not specify what the "something" was. But it sounded exciting, and I eagerly awaited the onrush of some blissful experience. However, the only thing that happened was that my arms ached and eventually I wobbled into a loss of balance and came out of the pose.

The second day, we did that pose again, and this time I vowed to stay in it until "something happened." Expectantly, I scanned my body, watching and feeling for the first hint of something magical, different, special. Nothing happened, except that I noted with interest my own predilection for the new and the surprising. I saw clearly that inner child in me who is totally hooked on treats and surprises.

The tree pose was already part of my daily routine. But after the workshop, I amended it to the hands over head version. And every day, as I stood there on one leg, I waited once more for "something to happen." It must be twenty years now, and the young man with the dark eyes has gray hair now, like me, and still I stand on one leg, every morning, and hear his voice. And still I wait, half hoping that eventually, if I do it for long enough, "something will happen."

Maybe one day, before we both die, I shall ask him to reveal the secret. "Just out of interest," I shall say to him, "What was it that was supposed to happen?" (At which he'll probably look vague and reply "Huh?") But, of course, it really does not matter. The beautiful thing about a gift like that is that it is personalized to fit. Like the magic lamp that you rub to get wishes granted, it is a gift that can give you anything you want it to give. Anything you need.

Standing on one leg, watching carefully, scanning my inner horizon for the first glimpse of the "something," I was fully present, fully attentive. Like a sailor on watch on the ship's bridge, I have stood and watched, and in the course of watching I have noticed everything that passed through my mind and body in those moments—every feeling, every thought, every bodily sensation. And over the years, as I have stood and watched, I have learned a lot about what does pass through. That quality of attention, that time of deep watching, that is the gift. For it reveals us to ourselves. And if we watch ourselves deeply enough, and for long enough, then it is not only our selves that become revealed, but the whole Universe, of which our selves are but a fragment.

We are not simply fragments of the Universe in the sense that a piece of broken glass is a fragment of the whole vase. We are holographic fragments. In holography, as you probably know, objects are recorded and reproduced, using laser beams, in three-dimensional wholeness rather than on a flat surface. When the beam is directed again through the glass plate containing the holographic image, the image is projected several feet out into the air in front, as though it were real. You can walk around it and see it from all sides. This is a fascinating experience. But what I find most fascinating of all is that if you smash a holographic plate, any single fragment of that plate, when the laser beam is directed through it, will reflect, not a piece of the image, but the whole image. It will be a little fuzzier than it would be if you had the intact plate, but it will still contain the entire image, no matter how small the fragment.

And that is how we are, each one of us, holographic fragments of a huge and amazing Universe.

No matter who we are, no matter what age or sex, race or nationality, no matter what our occupation, our interests, our lifestyle, we are all fragments of this Universe which burst into being fifteen billion years ago and which has been steadily expanding, developing and complexifying ever since.

The raw material of which we are composed is the same raw material that was present then, albeit in a different form. And when we die, that same raw material will continue to exist, to the end of time, endlessly circulating and re-circulating and changing shape but remaining a part of the whole, a fragment of something so huge and vast and awesome that our minds cannot even comprehend its totality.

If you look around at the philosophies, histories and lifestyles of all the various cultures of the world, you will find that the most balanced, contented and well-adapted groups—and for that matter the most balanced, contented and well-adapted individuals—are those who, in some way, continue to incorporate this sense of belonging into their lives and folkways. It makes sense, if you think about it. If you maintain a constant awareness of being part of something larger than yourself, then you feel at home in your skin, at home in your place, amongst your people. When you feel that sense of belonging, that sense of identification with the place and the people around you, you treat the place and the people with love and respect. Any tribe of people which feels a deep sense of belonging in the world, does not trash, exploit or otherwise damage the world. If we love our homes, we take care of them; if we are proud of our automobiles, we do not scratch their paint; if we feel at home in our bodies, we do not abuse them, but live in them respectfully and gracefully.

In the modern Western world, as we know, there is so much distraction, so much noise and hype, so much to pull us away from our sense of deep belonging, that we can easily lose our equilibrium. We can be seduced by the consumer culture into forgetting our connection with whole web of life and mindlessly joining in the exploitation and gang rape of our larger body, the Earth, using up her resources at a much faster rate than she can possibly replace them. It is so easy to forget, so easy to get caught up in the rush and hassle of making a living, getting and spending, "keeping up." So in order to stay centered and balanced, in order to stay connected with our true natures, our deeper selves, we all need some kind of personal spiritual practice.

As we grow older, the physical changes in our bodies and the fear of approaching death can cause many of us to lose equilibrium. So at this time in our lives, in order to remain balanced and centered, our spiritual practice becomes particularly important.

This does not necessarily mean going to church, though that may be the form it could take for some people. Neither does it mean that we have to twist our bodies into yoga postures or do tai chi in the park every morning, although both are fine options. In fact, it may not involve any change in our outer activities at all, but merely an inner change of emphasis on what is important and what is not.

Those who have followed some sort of regular practice over many years may actually find it diminishing as they get into their third age. We may notice ourselves spending less time in meditation, for example, or deciding to stay home instead of going to church services or workshops or spiritually focused group meetings. This need not be a cause for alarm or self-chastisement. For it may well be that our practices have become so much a part of our lives that we no longer need to devote as much time to deliberate cultivation of them. Our whole day may have become a meditation of sorts. Our spiritual lives have now become so important to us that all our outward activities now have an inward spiritual component of which we are often aware.

On the other hand, there are many of us entering our third age who have been so busy and preoccupied up till now that we have found insufficient time to devote to spiritual practice of any kind. So for us, it is important, now, to find ourselves a suitable vehicle for awakening that spiritual aspect.

Most of us find ourselves intuitively drawn towards one particular practice. However, as we grow and change in the course of our lives, we may find that different forms are appropriate at different stages. Or we may enjoy exploring, sampling, trying out different practices, seeing if they fit.

Here, again, is the question of balance. On the one hand, we could spend our whole lives shopping around and never settle with one practice. Many people use this as a way of avoiding the inner work of self-confrontation that spiritual practice inevitably entails. Buddhist psychologist Jack Kornfield gives some useful advice about what he calls "taking the one seat." He points out that if we do a little of one kind of practice and a little of another, it is a bit like digging many shallow wells instead of one deep one. By chopping and changing our practice too much we can sneakily avoid our deeper issues.[1]

On the other hand, we are not static creatures. Just as our bodies change, and the clothes in our wardrobes gradually change over the years, so do we grow and change inwardly as well. And different practices may be needed at different stages of our lives. There are things we can learn from group-type practices that we could never have learned from practicing alone, and there are physical insights that our bodies can attain from, say, yoga, that they could never attain from pure sitting meditation.

Furthermore, we may unwittingly find ourselves in a situation where remaining with the practice is not in our best interests. This is a particular problem of the "guru scene" where we see examples of people being emotionally and even physically damaged by remaining steadfastly involved with spiritual teachers who have fallen prey to the temptations of power, sexual or financial exploitation, or substance addiction. In cases like this, we need to know when it is time to get out. Our commitment is to our own spiritual growth and to the practice which will support that, not to the teachers themselves, in all their human fallibility. (And lest we assume that this is a problem only of Eastern traditions, it happens occasionally in Christian churches of all denominations as well.)

It pays us to remember that in any setting where people come together in groups to focus their attention together on one purpose, whether it be a football game, a political rally or a religious or spiritual ritual, a huge vortex of energy can be created. This energy can, like fire, be used for good or evil intent. The raw group energy present in a revivalist meeting is not essentially different in nature from that produced at one of Hitler's rallies or a Klan burning. It is what we do with it that matters. Group energy can transform consciousness, heal the sick, win a match, start a war. So in general, the practices which involve groups are the ones which carry the greatest dangers. They may also carry the greatest potential for learning and growth, since group experiences can carry such a powerful charge and imprint themselves upon us so vividly.

Another aspect of this is that we are by nature herd animals and learn well in groups. Whenever I want to relax my body quickly, I have only to tune in to the forty-year old memory of the voice of my very first yoga teacher quietly inviting each muscle to relax.

I remember, too, the atmosphere in the room where a hundred people sat in silence in front of a certain venerable spiritual teacher. In that setting, one had only to have the intention to meditate and the mind would drop effortlessly into it, like a stone into a clear, deep pool.

There is no mystery in the mechanics of this. By a process the scientists call entrainment, our brain's electrical rhythms tend to come into a synchronized pattern with those of another.

No matter how powerful our group experiences are, we also need ways of anchoring ourselves, every day, wherever we are, in that reality of being a fragment of the whole. So we need to develop some kind of individual, solitary practice also. Furthermore, no group practice is going to make any difference to us unless we are participating in it fully and consciously, in every moment, at an individual level. In that sense, I suppose you could say that all practice is, in fact, individual.

My own practice of choice is the Buddhist practice of mindfulness meditation, also known as Vipassana. This is the practice of sitting quietly and observing, without comment or judgment, the flow of content as it passes through the mind.[2]

Mindfulness meditation is rather like sitting on a railway platform, watching the trains go by but not catching any of them. A steady stream of thoughts, pictures, words, ideas, feelings, plans, memories is forever passing through, and most of the time we get caught up in the content of it. We get on a train, ride it a few stations, jump on another, ride it somewhere else, and so on, ever restless, ever on the move. The mind, Buddhists say, is like a monkey, leaping from branch to branch. It is pointless to try and change the nature of a monkey, and equally pointless to try and stop the mind from doing its thing. That is its sole purpose, to generate thoughts, feelings, ideas, etc., and to explore them, play with them, use them. As John O' Donohue says

> *Thoughts are the furniture of the mind. They are the*
> *echoes and pictures that hold your world together.*[3]

In mindfulness meditation, we do not chastise the mind for its preoccupation with thoughts, we simply learn to detach from the flow. We learn to observe the content as it passes through, without becoming swept up in it. In doing so, we eventually become able to penetrate beyond the level of thoughts, worries and preoccupations, and begin to see the Bigger Picture, the vast and wondrous Universe and how we fit into it.

Once we get into a practice like this, our own personal "stuff" inevitably starts emerging. Old wounds may surface, painful memories, dysfunctional patterns, childhood resentments—the works. The trick here is still the same—not to get caught up in the content, but simply to allow and accept. It is as though we bow respectfully to every item the mind throws up, without feeling the need to hug it to our bosom.

It seems paradoxical that while most people who engage in some kind of personal spiritual practice have a clear sense of the journey, of growing, changing, moving forward, at the same time there is a feeling of circularity. When the same issues come up again and again, it is easy to feel as though one is going in circles, getting nowhere.

In fact, if we could map our journey, it might look like a spiral, a combination of forward momentum and endless circularity. If you have looked carefully at the way you deal with those old familiar issues each time you re-encounter them, you may have noticed that with each encounter they are more deeply understood—and, what is even more important, more deeply accepted. For at the end of all our journeying, as the poet T.S. Eliot so beautifully said, we find ourselves at home with ourselves, back in that familiar place, but knowing it fully for the first time.[4] That is the reward of elderhood. So yes, we change, and no, we don't. The true change, the ultimate spiritual transformation, is not that we become something else, something "better." It is that we shift and grow in our understanding and acceptance of ourselves, and of each other, just as we are. We learn to accept ourselves and our fellow beings without judgment, blame or attachment.

Of course, few of us ever arrive at that perfect place of acceptance and non-attachment. But it really does not matter, for the truly important thing is the journey. And for the elderwoman, the honoring of her soul, the body's pilot on this amazing journey, is one of the most significant things she can do.

(I still wonder what that "something" was that was supposed to happen to me if I stood on one leg long enough. Perhaps it was this very realization of the importance of the journey rather than the destination.)

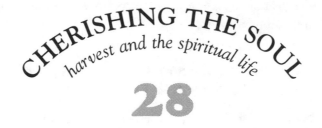

CHERISHING THE SOUL
harvest and the spiritual life
28

RENÉ DESCARTES, the seventeenth-century French philosopher and mathematician, whose concept of the mechanical, clockwork universe influenced the development of modern science, believed that the human soul resided in the tiny pineal gland, deep inside the brain. This notion of the soul residing in the body as some kind of appendage, rather than being the essence of who we are and the prime mover of our lives, has affected our culture ever since.

Though none of us, with our finite human minds, could ever comprehend the mysteries of the Universe, we can all theorize. So I like to think that if our physical selves are corpuscles of the physical Earth, then maybe our souls are corpuscles of the Earth soul. I see them as the individual expressions of that life energy which animates everything on Earth, and that, in turn, as part of a greater soul—let's call it the soul of the Universe. That soul of the Universe, which encompasses all of existence, is, of course, what some people know as God. When a fragment of this whole, an individual soul, temporarily takes bodily form, it enables the soul to be experienced by others, even though it can never be directly seen.

The soul of another, as we perceive it, is like a pure essence. It is something way beyond the creases and folds and protuberances of physical form or of individual character. It is something everlasting which we can neither describe nor explain and yet can feel and sense. It is that which we meet when we gaze into the depths of someone's eyes. When someone nears death, it is that which becomes more and more strongly present in the room and which departs as the last breath is taken, so that what is left now feels like a mere husk. And if we are open to it, it is also that which can suddenly and unexpectedly reach out to touch us from beyond the grave, filling our hearts with inexplicable joy, despite grief about our loved one's departure. In that second, we know that the person we loved is not lost to us at all, and never will be.

John O'Donohue says:

> As your body ages and gets weaker, your soul is in fact
> getting richer, deeper and stronger.[1]

In the final days of her life, my mother's face lost the plump and rounded softness she had inherited from her mother and the bony, aquiline features of her father began to show through more and more. She was revealing her skeleton, her essential physical structure. It was as though her soul was slowly undressing. It reminds me of those old ghost movies where the ghost is invisible until it picks up a book or puts on a scarf. When we undress from our physical form and cast our bodies off, our ever present souls become invisible to those around us.

It is hardly surprising then, that as we age, and draw closer to the moment of that last undressing, the soul becomes gradually more significant to us than the body. The wellbeing of the soul becomes the key factor in our overall health. The sacred dimensions of ordinary life become increasingly important, overshadowing any need we may have had for material gain or profit.

In this final chapter of our lives, we must not only honor the existence of this soul—this essence and guiding force in ourselves and others—but also cherish it most lovingly. So let us look once again at those elderwoman principles that we have collected up, like seashells, on our journey through this book, and see how they apply to the cherishing of our souls and how they may be incorporated into the last act of our lives—our dying.

Here is our whole collection of twenty principles:

• simplicity • deep vision • passion • compassion • non-attachment • Earth-centeredness • comfort • connectedness • respect • creativity • delight • lightness • enoughness • heart-listening • peace and quiet • authenticity • responsibility • radical aliveness • acceptance of change • balance •

252

Simplifying, as we age, becomes not only a matter of managing with fewer possessions but of gradually shedding the ballast which ties us to this life, so that by the time we reach the end we shall have achieved the necessary lightness to let go of whatever remains, including the bodies in which these souls have dwelt, and merge back into that greater soul, the way a river rejoins the ocean. If we have managed to cultivate the art of non-attachment, we can retain our bonds of love without a feeling of clinging. Just as an autumn leaf falls effortlessly from the tree, we shall be able to let go, to accept that great, final change of a lifetime—the moment of death—with equanimity.

If we listen carefully to our inner selves, we discover that the craving to have and to get will gradually leave us. In its place, comes a feeling of satisfaction—of enoughness. In those last years, as our mobility lessens and we spend more and more time in contemplation, looking back on all our experiences and life-lessons, this process of life review yields up to us a richer and richer harvest of wisdom.

Just as we looked, in an earlier chapter, at the food, vitamins and minerals we need to maintain physical and mental health in our third age, so we need to remember now all the things upon which our souls feed. The soul nutrients we must give ourselves now are things like peace and quiet, comfort, time and space in which to mull over our memories, and as many opportunities as possible for the types of spiritual practice that will lead us naturally into a feeling of completion.

We also need to prepare for our death, physically, mentally and emotionally, in the same way that one prepares for childbirth and with just as much attention to detail. In the same way that the best-made birth plans may be swept aside at the last minute by sudden emergency, like needing a C-section, death, too, may be sudden, messy and undignified, with loved ones far away. But we can still plan. For all such planning aids us in coming to terms with the inescapable truth that death will one day happen.[2]

I used to imagine that when I became very old, there would be a final mad dash to get everything finished to my satisfaction in time for the bell. After all, I have always been one of those people who tends to leave things till the last minute. And when I was in my early fifties, I still had a long mental list of all the things I wanted to complete in my lifetime—a huge agenda of treats not yet sampled, tasks not yet tackled, glories not yet won. I lived in terror of being called away too soon—of dying with a book half written, an attic unsorted, letters unsent, and a laundry hamper full of dirty linen. I thought I would have to force myself to slow down, to accept the frustration of not being able to complete all the things I wanted to do in my lifetime. But I was still looking at my third age with mid-life eyes

What made a difference, by the time I reached my middle sixties, was the discovery that nature herself, if we listen, gives us many of the prompts we need. The third age has its own curriculum. And part of that curriculum is learning to notice how sweet and elegant and totally trustworthy is the system of communication between our individual soul fragments and the great, universal soul of which they are a part. Just as we can, if we listen attentively, hear the wise words of a tree, so can we learn to read the messages which are all around and within us, every moment of our lives, instructing us what we need to do and when. This is a part of our heart-listening.

We do not need to figure out any of our major third age tasks with our intellects. They happen automatically—if we give them space and encourage them; if we see them as natural, rather than feeling guilty or resentful about them. The things our soul needs to do will get done. The things our mind imagines we want to do are really unimportant. And the older we get, the more we feel the truth of that. Desires become mere preferences. We may imagine that all the old plans and dreams are still there. But if we go within and look more carefully at them, we often find , to our surprise, that only the outer packaging remains. The contents have evaporated. For all they really were is unexamined leftovers from an earlier era.

An aunt of mine, now in her late eighties, informs me ruefully, every time I visit her, that she is "really lazy nowadays." Instead of all the gardening and sewing, knitting and preserving she used to do, she now spends most of her time sitting in a chair, unable to walk unaided because of problems in her legs. She refuses to accept my suggestion that sitting quietly in a chair at her age, "achieving" very little in an outward way, is a perfectly natural state of affairs. What I haven't the heart to tell her is that if she were to try tuning in to the vast world within her instead of the plastic world of TV, she might realize why her soul wants to sit still right now and thus be more comfortable with the whole process.

My mother, who had completed a crossword every day of her adult life, put her crossword book down a week or so before she died. She was still chatting brightly that day. The next day, she spoke less, and the day after that, less still.

The signs are always there. Just as animals know that a thunderstorm is approaching, we, too, can be effortlessly aware of where we are and what is coming next.

Ram Dass, in his book, *Still Here: Embracing Aging, Changing and Dying*, describes the way Tibetan monks and nuns are trained to guide a dying person through the process:

> *As the earth element leaves, your body will feel heavy. As the water element leaves, you will feel dryness. As the fire element leaves, you may feel cold. As the air element leaves, your outbreath will be longer than your inbreath. The signs are now here. Don't get lost in the detail. Don't cling to any of these phenomena. They are part of a natural process. Let your Awareness go free.*[3]

The ultimate take-home message I would like to leave you with is this notion of allowing our deepest nature to guide us rather than attempting to impose our willful agendas on the third age of our lives.

These elderwoman principles which we have collected are not so much tools whose use we have to master, like the tools of our heroic youth, but sieves into which we can put all the stuff of our lives and watch the bits we no longer need fall through the holes.

Our creativity naturally turns towards handcrafting our elderwoman lives—if we let it. Deep vision and compassion naturally arise within us—if we get out of the way and allow them to. The Earth calls us, reminding us that we belong to it, singing to us the song of our own clay beings, helping us remember that we shall rest into it again, five, ten, twenty, thirty years from now. Comfort calls us: my grandmother's favorite old maroon cardigan with the little metal buttons that she wore over everything, summer and winter; my friend Jenny's sweat pants and sneakers; the thick drink of eggs and milk my great-grandfather used to ask for again and again when he was ninety-six and had no teeth to chew with; my aunt's brand-new electric recliner chair with more controls than a helicopter.

Heart-listening enables us to sieve out the oughts and shoulds and advertising; passion calls us to the issues that really matter—both to ourselves and to the world—and balance guarantees that we shall have what we need in all the right amounts. Above all, a commitment to radical aliveness sieves out all negativity by taking us to a place where everything that happens to us, whether pleasant or painful, is equally and wonderfully OK and delight is guaranteed.

Connectedness sieves out loneliness, isolation and alienation, and the cultivation of respect teaches us to sieve out the kinds of judgment which might also set us apart and alienate us from the wider world of human and non-human companions.

Responsibility empowers us. With our sense of responsibility as elders, we need no longer feel useless, spare or forgotten. We have a vital role to play. Even in our dying, we play it, for in our demonstration of our own authenticity and the acceptance of our aging and death we are setting an example that helps free the world from its collective fears and denials.

In our third age, if we embrace all these principles, we shall not have to struggle to live our lives. Instead, we can simply allow *them* to live *us*.

So cherishing the soul means turning the agenda of our earlier lives on its head. Now it is time to listen, to attend, to let the Earth-soul, of which we are a part, steadily draw these individual fragments back into itself. To feel the Earth being lived deeply through us instead of imagining that we live on top of it, like so many sprinkles on a birthday cake.

This, not fame nor fortune, is our ultimate achievement.

If we can let go of our attachments, while retaining and deepening our love, then those who love us will find it easier to let us move on. Our acceptance of aging and our openness about death will make their own roles easier. To live as an elderwoman is a triumph. To die as an elderwoman, an even greater one. At the end, there is no agenda other than to be.

If there is something which you are able to do, then do it, and it will be enough. If all that you are able to do is to care, then caring is enough. When the time comes to let go of everything, even caring, then let go. And as that great elderwoman of a long ago time, Julian of Norwich said, "All shall be well. All manner of thing shall be well."

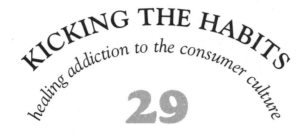

KICKING THE HABITS
healing addiction to the consumer culture
29

WE ARE NEARLY at the end of this book, so let's take a look back at the path we have walked together.

In the first section, we looked at the seasons of a woman's life and at the bridge of menopause which leads into the third age. We then went on to consider our relationships to the earthy things—the soil, our homes, other people and other creatures, and the planet Earth herself.

Next, we looked at the air element and that whole aspect of growing old which I refer to as "lightening," and then at the fiery aspects of our lives, the personal and political passions which fire us up, and the concerns of our hearts and hearths.

Following that, we pondered a while on the watery, flowing element in our lives, seeing life itself as a flowing, ever changing river, and looking, too, at the ways in which time flows.

Finally, we have looked at balancing the elements of our lives to create a roundly satisfying, productive, healthy and serene old age, and at how we might approach the door of death.

In this wide-ranging discussion, few of the ideas I have presented are new, but I believe that, connected in this way, they form a useful guide to living a meaningful life in one's third age. There will be much I have left out. But that is OK. I cannot write the definitive book on who or what the elderwoman is, for she is a work-in-progress, a collective creation. The creation of her belongs not to me but to us all. And it belongs not just now but to the future.

One day, I hope, almost every post-menopausal woman you meet will be an elderwoman. It will come to be expected that every elderwoman, in

257

her own way, discharges her responsibility of caring for the Earth, for the soil, for all other creatures, for the future of generations yet unborn. It will be taken for granted that she has wisdom to offer, vision to lend to any worthwhile project which captures her attention, and a personal lifestyle of simplicity and delight. Unfortunately, we have quite a way to go before that happens. So there is many a fully fledged elderwoman of today who finds herself somewhat alone in her beliefs, ideas and practices.

Someone who has reached this point will probably have left behind many of the more crass and dysfunctional aspects of the mainstream culture. But just as we find that the farther away from the parking lot we walk, the fewer people are on the trail, so it is with this. We may even be seen as oddities by some of the people around us. An elderwoman who lives simply, gives things away, cares about the soil, is fanatical about recycling, writes letters to her local paper, likes to walk or ride a bike instead of taking her car, dresses for comfort rather than style, meditates, boycotts unethical trade practices and stays away from supermarkets and out of McDonalds might perhaps stand out from the crowd as unusual—even eccentric.

Sometimes others find this inspiring. Sometimes it makes them feel guilty. They may even put subtle pressure on her to become more like them. Though they admire her lifestyle, their perception of her as different may be subtly alienating for her at times. Occasionally, she may find herself going along with things she neither wants nor enjoys in order to feel less alienated—and then feeling cross with herself afterwards.

Before I leave you, therefore, I wanted to include this chapter on the difficulties of changing behaviors which, while normal to the statistical majority, may, nevertheless, be dysfunctional and addictive. It is not always thought of in this way, but like Chellis Glendinning, I am convinced that the average Western lifestyle, with its shallow, sensationalist media, its fast food and consumer values is in many ways an addict's lifestyle.[1] We can think of the elderwoman as someone who has recovered and who, by her example, gently encourages others to do the same. So I will briefly mention three common stumbling blocks to recovery. The first is peer pressure.

Everyone knows how difficult it is for the drug addict to come out of a rehab center and go back on the street without falling back into the ways of the group. We all know how difficult it is for someone newly teetotal to go to the bar and drink mineral water. But no one talks much about the peer group pressures that lock us into almost every other facet of our lives in the consumer society. No one talks about peer pressure to watch TV and know who the latest "stars" are, have the radio going all the time, drink coffee, waste electricity, live on credit, shop, travel by car (preferably late model) instead of public transport, follow fashions, use disposables or eat junk food, but it is there, just the same. Our Western society has a mass addiction to its way of life. And the pushers are working hard to make sure that the addiction spreads worldwide. The tobacco industry, for example, with its sales waning in the U.S. and western Europe, now spends millions on advertising campaigns in the Middle East and in eastern Europe, deliberately targeting young teenagers. Consumerism is wreaking havoc in traditional cultures, all over the world.

So if recovery is our aim, then we need to acknowledge that we cannot dissolve that addiction by pure intent and willpower alone. We need to call on what the Alcoholics Anonymous people call a "higher power." However, this higher power we call on is, in fact, a deeper part of ourselves—the part that knows, intuitively, what is best for our bodies, our souls and our Earth.

If we find ourselves moving away from many of the interests and pursuits of our mainstream culture, either by conscious choice or because by now, in the process of becoming elderwomen, we are simply outgrowing them, then we may find—as recovering addicts do—that our recovery has certain effects on our relationships with others. Families and friends, colleagues—even acquaintances—like us to remain as we are; they prefer that we should appear consistent, predictable and unchanging . While on the one hand humans crave novelty and excitement, on the other hand we fear it and shrink from change. The only way we can handle change is if we ourselves are controlling it. But when others change, it scares us. So whenever we begin to do things differently in our own lives we can expect some resistance from the folks around us, and the more definite or permanent the change appears to be, the greater the resistance.

In time, of course, adaptation happens. Human beings are highly adaptable, which is probably the secret of our proliferation as a species. Just as we adjust eventually to even the most heart-wrenching bereavements, to life after war, disaster, holocaust and permanent injury, so do we adjust, after a little time, to the changes we at first resisted. When we ourselves make changes, therefore, we can reassure ourselves that others' resistance will give way eventually to their acceptance of the new status quo.

In kicking cultural habits, as in other addictions, the second stumbling-block is the problem of re-calibration.

One of the ways we avoid pain is to try and replace it with something pleasurable, the way children are given candy to cover the taste of unpleasant medicine. To assuage the pain of loneliness, the despair of meaninglessness, and the loss of the sacred in their lives, people turn to food for which they are not truly hungry, to drink for which they are not really thirsty, to drugs, to cigarettes. Thus we train our bodies to override the normal signals that would tell us when we have had enough. In the most advanced cases of addiction, "enough" only comes when the point of satiation has been reached. The drunk falls into a stupor, the binge-eater rushes to the bathroom to purge. After a while, the body gives up and forgets how to send the "enough" signals as well as how to interpret them. I have worked with anorexic women whose addiction to the high of lightness, born out of the pain of inhabiting a normal, heavy body in a normal, troublesome world, has caused their organisms to forget completely the sensations of hunger or of its appeasement. They have to re-calibrate their systems by learning, all over again, how to eat, and how much.

In the same way, heroin addicts, whose bodies have re-set themselves to interpret the state of addiction as their normal baseline, have to re-calibrate by learning how to live without the drug and enjoy the everyday highs of normal life.

After fifty or more years of living in a society in which the enough point never seems to be reached, it can take an act of will, at first, to re-calibrate ourselves by establishing this sense of enoughness in our own lives, whether as regards food, consumer goods, excitement or anything else. This second stumbling-block forms, for many of us, a crucial part of our spiritual practice.

The third stumbling-block is the discovery of underlying pain.

Almost all the addicts I have ever known, whether addicted to drugs, alcohol, bingeing and vomiting, gambling, sensation, shopping, intensity of emotion, sex or whatever, have discovered that when the addiction is taken away, there are painful feelings to face, which the addiction had been masking.

It was, in many cases, the pain of these feelings and the attempt to avoid them that began the addiction in the first place. No matter how long the addiction lasts, feelings will sit there patiently, biding their time, and there they are, waiting to be faced, when the addiction ends.

In the same way, getting out from under the addictive habits of the industrial consumer culture brings an awareness of the problems which that culture has been unable to face. For this mechanism which operates at an individual level also operates, I believe, at a group level. Our whole society is hiding itself in its addictions and the problems it could not face are waiting patiently to be acknowledged and tackled. Therefore, one of our most painful tasks, as elderwomen, if we want our society as a whole to kick its habits, is to allow ourselves fully to feel the feelings which crowd in when the chattering stops, the electronic babble is turned off, and all is quiet. We need to allow ourselves to feel the despair that hangs like a dark cloud over our modern, polluted world. For until enough of us have felt it, acknowledged it, honored it, there will not be enough energy in our society to do the work that needs to be done to clean the world up.

You know how, when there is a large and difficult task to do, one tends to sit and read a book and hope it will all go away? We put off the moment of decision to grab that broom or that paintbrush, to get out all the receipts and start working out the taxes, to clean out the cupboards. Just one more cup of coffee and I'll start. Tomorrow, I'll start. When I have more energy, then I'll start. Meanwhile, we sit in a kind of paralysis. It is like the weariness that keeps us sitting in the chair way past bedtime. Our addictions serve to cover up the communal fear and despair that we all feel, underneath. But until we dissolve the addictions, uncover the fear and despair that is sitting there, and allow ourselves to feel and express it, we have no power or energy. For what is happening, of course, is that our energy is being used to maintain our defenses against the things we do not want to face.

It is like the grief and loss that we feel when we lose someone or something precious to us. If we do not allow ourselves to feel it and express it, we can never get past it and move on. Unfelt, unexpressed pain turns to depression, shutting us down, blanking us out, sapping our power and strength.

As Joanna Macy says:

> *Just as grief-work is a process by which bereaved persons unblock their numbed energies by acknowledging and grieving the loss of a loved one, so do we all need to unblock our feelings about our threatened planet and the possible demise of our species. Until we do, our power of creative response will be crippled.*[2]

This is where mindfulness practice comes into its own. In Macy's words again:

> Most people are afraid that if you feel despair you're going
> to be stuck in it, you're going to be mired in it, or you
> might break apart. And so it's helpful to experience that
> feelings can come and go and that though our connection
> with the world brings pain, we're not the kind of objects
> that will break. Pain and despair come and go just like
> feelings of love, delight and empowerment.[3]

All through history, it has been the older women who come in with their sleeves rolled up at times of change and transition. It is older women who have traditionally been there, always, at the entrances and exits and difficult times of life, delivering babies, laying out the dead and ministering to the sick, the old and the infirm. And it is elderwomen, now, who will be in the forefront when it comes to kicking the addictive habits of the consumer culture, bringing our ailing Earth back into balance and birthing a new and gentler vision for humanity.

This task demands heroism, but not heroism in the sense of bold, brave acts that the whole world sees and applauds. The heroism of the elderwoman is a quiet, inner heroism which, as Macy suggests, can face unpalatable truths and go to the full depths of a profound despair, knowing that she is "not the kind of object that will break." And there is more, beyond that. For when she has allowed the full extent of her despair to be felt and understood, she needs to take yet another step. This is to stretch her compassionate heart to embrace even the possibility of the destruction of everything she knows and loves. Knowing that she can never leave the Earth, and will be part of it for eternity, no matter what, she surrenders to the future, even if that future is one composed only of wind and salt water, bare rock, barren soil and sand. Whatever the future is, she cannot but be there. We shall all be there, whether we like it or not, reduced, once more, to our fundamental clay.

It is out of that total acceptance, that total detachment from outcomes—if we can ever achieve it—that we do our best and most passionate work. So that is the final habit the elderwoman has to kick, the habit of attachment to the outcomes of her actions—of anyone's actions. And it takes true heroism to kick that one!

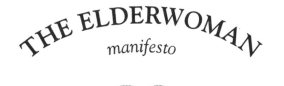

THE ELDERWOMAN
manifesto

30

WHEN THE last few remaining men and women of my mother's generation are all gone, there will be no one left alive who remembers horse-drawn carriages in the streets.

When I and my generation are gone, who will remember the smell of my grandmother's kitchen and the taste of my great-aunt's homemade elderberry wine?

In another thirty years, how many people still alive will remember how nice it was to have all your phone calls answered by a live person, to have a bank teller who knew your name, to get away to a place where no phones ever ring, and to be able to buy buttons or picture hooks loose instead of in packets of five or ten (when you needed six or twelve).

Just as heirloom varieties of vegetables are being lost in this modern world of seed patenting, hybridization and genetic manipulation, so are many of the valuable ideas, methods and values of yesterday being lost from contemporary memory.

We, the elderwomen, are the seed-savers.

It is up to us to ensure that the true treasures of our culture are preserved for future use. Just as my grandmother used to salt down beans for the winter, we, too, have to preserve, in our daily lives, things which we know to be deeply nourishing to the human body and soul and work to throw out things which we know to be destructive and harmful to ourselves, our loved ones, our communities or Earth herself.

But rather than attempting to turn back the clock, let us move forward, using every ounce of knowledge, wisdom, creativity and skill at our disposal to help construct a world which incorporates the best of the past with the achievements of the present and the vast potential of the future, a world which is based, for the first time in history, on the perfect balance and integration of the yin and the yang; the masculine and the feminine; the body, the mind, the heart, the soul and the spirit.

So what each of us needs, as we embark on this journey through the third age, is a medicine bundle, filled with the fragrant memories of all that is best about earlier, less frenetic ages, and with the seeds of all the wholesome and nourishing things which our world is in danger of forgetting—things like peace and quiet, the space between, the nothing which lends significance to whatever it frames, human-sized walking places, community, networks of grassroots economies, heart-to-heart interaction, places with centers, and simplicity in all its forms.

Finally, let each of us place, in her medicine bundle, the twenty principles of the elderwoman. Let us vow to

1. Embrace simplicity in every way we can

2. Use our deep vision to see beyond the illusions of the world

3. Nurture and express our passion

4. Temper our passion with compassion

5. Strive for the goal of non-attachment

6. Maintain Earth-centeredness

7. Celebrate comfort

8. Seek connectedness

9. Show respect towards all beings and ourselves

10. Use our creativity to handcraft our lives

11. Revel in the sense of delight

12. Enjoy the increasing lightness of aging

13. Remember to seek the point of enoughness

14. Practice heart-listening

15. Ensure our own peace and quiet and encourage others to appreciate theirs

16. Remember the importance of authenticity in all that we are and do

17. Take our share of responsibility for the healing of life on Earth

18. Meet each moment with radical aliveness

19. Accept the inevitability of change

20. Maintain balance in our own lives and work for a better balance in the world

Let each one of us use and live these principles, to the very best of her ability and find every possible opportunity to introduce them into the world around us.

We may not be able to change the world overnight. But even if only half us become elderwomen, we'll do it in a generation.

Let's go for it.

EPILOGUE
in praise of rose hips

LIKE MY grandmother, I love roses. A sweet, harmless interest for an old woman like me. But as well as gardening, I also do a lot of abstract thinking. I ponder on the symbolism of things, and rap about it with anyone who cares to join me. So I have been pondering about roses.

Unlike people, roses probably do not consider themselves as having a purpose in life. But if a rose bush did have a mission, I expect its greatest sense of achievement would come from creating, not just a whole lot of beautiful flowers, but the grand array of round, red rose hips which come after them.

Rose hips, as you know, are a concentrated source of vitamin C, the vitamin which does so much to protect our immune systems and shield us from illness. They are also very lovely objects in their own right. They are smooth and glowing, each one compact and complete in itself

I often think of the elderwoman as a kind of rose hip. Perhaps because my grandmother, my elderly aunts and many of the older women I saw around me as a child all had the round face and rosy cheeks so typical of the English West Country region from which I spring.

These old women, in their differing ways, were storehouses of wisdom. They knew how to make bread and cakes and wine, and how to grow walnut-sized loganberries and foot-long runner beans without the use of any artificial fertilizers. They made clotted cream from milk, hats from pieces of felt and wonderful garments from the bargain remnants they bought at end-of-season sales.

They were comfortable with the mysteries of life and death and knew all the rules for leading a good and moral existence. And for every occasion they had a wise saying, a witty ditty or a suitable song.

The wisdom of the elders is the vitamin C of traditional human communities. It protects them from attack by alien forces and from being swept away by the flood of new and untested ideas or destroyed by the cancer of internal conflict.

Unfortunately, in our youth-obsessed culture, where speed, glamour, fame and material success have become more important than reflective quiet, inner beauty, respect and the riches of the soul, few elders have been listened to of late. Their slower, more thoughtful voices tend to be drowned out by the contemporary clamor and their natural conservatism is often seen as an obstacle to growth and progress, like an ancient tree in the path of a bulldozer.

Many of yesterday's elderly were further disempowered by their natural reluctance to use the information technology by which so much cross-pollination of modern thinking takes place. So they were sidelined, and left to amuse themselves as best they could in the ever lengthening years of their old age.

Elders of both genders suffered from this sidelining effect, but I think the women suffered more from it than the men, since women so often internalize modern society's abhorrence of aging and its overvaluing of youth. Unlike men, women have suffered, as they aged, from an increasing sense of invisibility, their faces rarely reflected back to them in the media.

This brings me back to roses.

Roses grow in our modern gardens in an ever increasing variety of shapes, shades and sizes. We welcome the buds; we revel in the flowers. But when the petals fall, that's the end. A rosebud is beautiful, and the unfurling rose is an object of sensuous delight to eye and nose. But fading, falling petals, like wrinkles, drooping breasts and graying hair, are something our society has abhorred, up till now. We have been in the habit of deadheading our roses before the rose hips had a chance to ripen. Rose hips had nothing of value to offer—or so we foolishly supposed.

However, all that is changing. The emerging generations of aging women will not let themselves be sidelined like their predecessors. Once they have gotten through grieving for their fallen petals, and their natural energy begins to return, they will start noticing that new rose hip swelling in their hearts and begin to nurture and to cherish it. They will stand tall and proud, daring anyone to take clippers to their sturdy stems.

With the wisdom they have collected, from all those years of thinking, reading, talking, processing and transforming, I believe these elderwomen are going to do wonders for the immune systems of their communities.

Vitamin C has been known to work miracles of healing. It is about to do so again, on a bigger scale than we have ever seen.

So stand by for the twenty-first-century elderwoman. She is on her way.

Notes

Introduction

1. Marian Van Eyk McCain, *Transformation through Menopause* .
2. Carl Gustav Jung, *Collected Works*, Vol 8, paras 784–787.
3. Grizel Luttman-Johnson, "Old" (unpublished, ©1999).
4. Florida Scott-Maxwell, *The Measure of My Days*. In the form of an occasional diary, this book has become a classic, exploring the inner world of aging and the outer world as seen through the eyes of a woman in her eighties.
5. Grizel Luttman-Johnson, "Old"

Chapter 1. The Stages of Womanhood

1. Barbara Walker, *The Crone: Woman of Age, Wisdom and Power*, pp.24–25. Walker's book is a must-read for anyone interested in the history of attitudes to old women under patriarchy. (warning—it can arouse strong feelings of grief and rage).
2. Esther Harding, *Woman's Mysteries Ancient and Modern*. Harding, a pupil of Carl Jung, has done extensive research on the symbolism of the moon in both ancient and modern life.
3. Barbara Walker, *The Crone*, p.142

Chapter 2. The Transition

1. Ann Mankowitz's book, *Change of Life: A Psychological Study of Dreams and the Menopause* illustrates the menopause process through the dreams of one woman, recorded over time and discussed in therapy.
2. William Bridges, *Transitions: Making Sense of Life's Changes*. The wisdom in this little book can be applied to any type of major change in one's life

Chapter 3. Life as an Elderwoman

1. Alan Chinen, *In the Ever After: Fairy Tales and the Second Half of Life*, p.152. The stories in this book come from all over the world, each illustrating one or more of the developmental tasks of aging. Chinen has a Jungian and transpersonal perspective.
2. Ibid.
3. Paul Ray and Sherry Anderson, *The Cultural Creatives: How 50 Million People Are Changing the World*. www.culturalcreatives.org When you think you are alone in your ideas, this book is a cheering reminder that there are millions who share your beliefs and values.
4. Chinen, *In the Ever After*, p.125.

Chapter 4. The Dirt Beneath Our Feet

1. John O'Donohue, *Anam Cara*, p.94. A beautiful, lyrical book from this deep thinking, deep feeling, slow-speaking theologian from the west of Ireland. Also available as a tape set.

Chapter 5. Planet Earth

1. Paul Shepard, *The Only World We've Got*. One of the brilliant minds of our times, Paul Shepard died in 1996. He wrote with a richness of ideas and images in every paragraph.
2. Ibid., p.xx.

Chapter 6. Living Where We Live

1. Clare Cooper Marcus, *House as a Mirror of Self: Exploring the Deeper Meaning of Home*, p.247. A fascinating look at the way we express ourselves by our choice of living spaces and the way we furnish and decorate them.
2. Christopher Alexander, *A Pattern Language*, p387. Alexander and his colleagues compiled this book primarily for architects, hoping that it would inspire them to consider the human needs of the people for whom they were designing. It should be compulsory reading for anyone who is thinking of building, renovating or designing human habitat of any kind.
3. Ibid.

Chapter 7. Sharing the Earth Space

1. J. Allen Boone, *Kinship With All Life*. This charming little classic has been reprinted and is still easily available.
2. D.H.Lawrence, *Complete Poems*.
3. Brian Swimme and Thomas Berry, *The Universe Story*, p.103. In this book, all our scientific knowledge about the origins of the Earth is retold in the form of a story—the true story of creation.
4. Barbara Walker, *The Woman's Dictionary of Symbols and Sacred Objects*, p.247. A useful reference book for anyone interested in symbolism.
5. Lyn White Jnr., "The Historical Roots of our Ecologic Crisis" quoted in Warwick Fox, *Towards a Transpersonal Ecology*, p.6.

Chapter 8. The Handcrafted Life

1. See note 1 in Chapter 6.

Chapter 9. The Pure Joy of Simplicity

1. Leonard Koren, *Wabi-Sabi: for Artists, Designers, Poets and Philosophers*.

Chapter 10. The Other Side of the Mountain

1. Helen Luke's book, *Old Age, Journey into Simplicity* is presumably written for both women and men, although the literary characters she uses to illustrate it— such figures as Ulysses and Shakespeare's Prospero from *The Tempest*—are all male. She writes poignantly of the later life task of letting go of the ego-driven activities of one's middle years and resting into a life of simple ordinariness.

Notes

Chapter 11. Living Simply
1 Jared Diamond, *The Third Chimpanzee: The Evolution and Future of the Human Animal.*

Chapter 12. The Space Between
1. Lao Tzu, *Tao Te Ching*, XI: 27.
2. Karen Kingston, *Creating Sacred Space with Feng Shui*, p.231. Karen's best-known book is probably *Clear Your Clutter With Feng Shui*—a little book which has inspired many people to create more space in their environments and feel much better for doing so.
3. David Steindl-Rast, *A Listening Heart*, p.67. A small volume of inspirational essays from this Benedictine monk whose mission has been to build bridges between the various wisdom traditions, particularly Buddhism and Christianity.

Chapter 13. Traveling Light
1. T.H. Holmes and R.H. Rahe, "The social readjustment rating scale," (*Journal of Psychosomatic Research, 11,* 1967), pp.213-218.

Chapter 14. Keeper of the Flame
1. Hesiod, *Theogeny*, 454 ff. XXIX. "To Hestia" (ll. 1–6).
2. Rabbi Schachter-Shalomi, *From Age-ing to Sage-ing*. p.144.

Chapter 15. Blood
1. An academic, cross-cultural study of the way aging affects the roles of men and women in various cultures may be found in David Guttman's book *Reclaimed Powers: Towards a New Psychology of Men and Women in Later Life.*
2. Joel Wilbush, "Climacteric Expression & Social Context" in *Maturitas* 4 n.33 (1982), p.203.
3. Carolyn Heilbrun, *The Last Gift of Time: Life After Sixty*, p.11.
4. Ibid., p.209.
5. Jean Shinoda Bolen, *Goddesses in Everywoman.*
6. ——— *Goddesses in Older Women.*
7. Heilbrun, *The Last Gift*, p.67–68.

Chapter 16 Fire in the Belly
1. Mary F. Belenky et al, *Women's Ways of Knowing: The Development of Self, Voice, and Mind.*
2. James Hillman, *The Force of Character*, pp.5–6.
3. Thich Nhat Hanh, *Being Peace*, pp.63–64. One of the many slim volumes of inspiration by this Vietnamese monk who espouses what he calls "engaged Buddhism."
4. Belenky, *Women's Ways of Knowing.*
5. Scott-Maxwell, *The Measure of My Days*, p. 3. (see Chapter 1, Note 3).

Chapter 17. Taking the Risk
1. Brian Swimme and Thomas Berry, *The Universe Story*, (see Chapter 7, Note 3).

2. Deepak Chopra, *Perfect Health*. This prolific author, an endocrinologist whose wisdom has transformed the lives of thousands, has re-awakened Western interest in Ayurvedic medicine.
3. Sandra Haldeman Martz (ed), *When I am an Old Woman I Shall Wear Purple: An Anthology of Short Stories and Poetry*. Foreword by Jenny Joseph, author of the poem which inspired the title.
4. Ruth Harriet Jacobs, *Be an Outrageous Older Woman*. A light-hearted book with lots of tips and ideas for enjoying the third age.
5. Naomi Wolf, *The Beauty Myth: How Images of Beauty are Used Against Women*, p.95.
6. Barbara McDonald and Cynthia Rich, *Look Me in the Eye: Old Women, Aging, and Ageism* These two were pioneers. Theirs was the book which first put the word 'ageist' into our vocabulary.

Chapter 18. Deconstructing
1. Theodore Roszak, *America the Wise*, p.11.
2. Ibid.

Chapter 19. The Juicy Life
1. Richard Moss, *The Black Butterfly*, p.275.

Chapter 20. Looking Upstream
1. Erik Erikson, *Childhood and Society*.
2. Eric Berne, *Games People Play: The Psychology of Human Relationships*. This was the first book to introduce what went on to become a whole discipline in its own right—Transactional Analysis—very popular in the 1970s.
3. Roberto Assagioli's book *Psychosynthesis* is the original text for this, but there are many other books which present his ideas in a very readable way, for example, Piero Ferrucci's *What We May Be: Techniques for Psychological and Spiritual Growth*.
4. Erik Erikson with J. Erikson and H. Kivnick, *Vital Involvement in Old Age*.
5. Carl Gustav Jung, *The Collected Works of C.G. Jung*. There are lots of things written specifically on this aspect of the "shadow," for example Robert Johnson's excellent little book *Owning Your Own Shadow*.
6. James Hillman, *The Force of Character*.
7. Schachter-Shalomi, From Age-ing to Sage-ing, pp.267–285.

Chapter 21. Looking Downstream
1. Jean Liedloff, *The Continuum Concept*.
2. Joseph Chilton Pearce. *Evolution's End: Claiming the Potential of Our Intelligence*. A psychologist, who has spent twenty years researching human intelligence and development. Pearce asserts that since the end of WW II, we have been systematically sabotaging our children's development (and therefore our future) and that this damage has reached critical and perhaps irreversible proportions. We do this through 1) contemporary hospital birthing techniques, which short-circuit natural mother–child bonding; 2) contemporary extended daycare and

premature schooling, which further weakens the parent–child bonding process, creates a traumatic feeling of abandonment, and disrupts natural development rhythms; and 3) television, which seriously impedes vital neurological development and kills creative play.

3. Robert Bly, *The Sibling Society*. Bly maintains that we have neglected our elders and abandoned our children to become a horizontal sibling society of adolescents attempting to raise each other.

Chapter 22. The Juice That Flows

1. In the United States, maquiladoras would most likely be called sweatshops. There are close to a million maquiladora workers in Mexico. Many of them are girls and young women from 14 to 20 years old. They work six days a week in grueling 10-hour shifts with few breaks. Working conditions are often hazardous, and industrial accidents and toxic exposures are common. On average, the workers earn between $0.80 and $1.25 an hour, and they often are unaware of their rights under Mexico's labor code.

    In addition, maquiladoras contribute little, if anything, to Mexico's development. In the name of job creation, the maquiladoras are exempted from paying taxes to their host country. Most maquiladora workers live in shantytowns that lack basic services such as water, sewage, or electricity.

    Furthermore, only 1 percent of the components for maquiladora products are made in Mexico, so the industry also doesn't help stimulate the local economy. One "contribution" the maquiladoras do make is pollution. Many maquiladoras do not comply with regulations for the safe disposal of hazardous wastes, which by law must be returned to the United States. (*Quote from the website of the American Friends Service Committee* <www.afsc.org/border/maquila.htm>)

2. Roszak, American the Wise, p.167.
3. Caz Challis, "I Always Knew I'd Be Old" (unpublished, © 2000).

Chapter 23. Flow as Absorption

1. Mihalyi Csikszentmihalyi, *Flow: the Psychology of Optimal Experience*. Professor Csikszentmihalyi's study was a huge and impressive one, involving eight thousand subjects from all walks of life. The phenomenon of flow was experienced in hundreds of different types of activity.

2. Roszak, American the Wise.

Chapter 24. Honoring Both Mother and Father

1. Ordained in 1961, Robert Fulghum was a part-time Unitarian minister from 1961 to 1985 in Washington. One of his favorite sermon and essay topics was the value of kindergarten rules. His essay on the subject circulated in the Unitarian community and eventually found its way into the workplace, the "Dear Abby" column, and even the *Congressional Record*. Finally, a literary agent read the work and contacted him. The essay, along with many of his other writings, became the bestseller entitled, *"All I Really Need to Know I Learned in Kindergarten."*

Chapter 25. Honoring the Body

1. Joe Dominguez and Vicki Robin, *Your Money Or Your Life: Transforming Your Relationship with Money and Achieving Financial Independence*.
2. In aiding ourselves to understand the hidden message of medical symptoms, it is interesting and useful to read the work of authors like Caroline Myss, who have made a study of this connection (see Bibliography for details of her book *Anatomy of the Spirit*).

Chapter 26. Cherishing the Body

1. See Chapter 17, note 2 on Deepak Chopra.
2. The foremost writer on Macrobiotics is Michio Kushi, whose wife, Aveline, supplies recipes to accompany his writings on how to balance one's nutritional intake according to the principles of yin and yang.
3. The notion of one's perfect diet being ordained by blood type is a fairly new one which has aroused a lot of interest. See Dr. D'Adamo's book *Eat Right for Your Type*. As a vegetarian who, according to Dr Adamo's theory, should be eating red meat, I have problems with it, but I know people who swear that it has helped them enormously.
4. For much of this information on osteoporosis I am indebted to Carol Leonard of Concord, NH, a certified midwife with twenty years experience in healthcare and co-author (with Elizabeth Davis) of *The Women's Wheel of Life*.
5. Sherwin Nuland, *How We Die: Reflection on Life's Final Chapter*. This is a typically "medical model" book, written in terms of wars and battles against disease, but interesting, and frankly informative about the way our bodies finally give out.
6. Nicholas Albery, Gil Eliot and Joseph Eliot, eds., *The New Natural Death Handbook*.
7. Lisa Carlson, *Caring for the Dead: Your Final Act of Love*, p.9.
   Explaining why she wrote the book, Lisa says: "After my husband John died, there was a lot of publicity (with my permission) about the fact that I had handled my own "arrangements." Hardly a week went by in the following year without a telephone call or letter from someone else involved in the plans surrounding a death. I also was asked to speak to church groups and classes on 'Death and Dying.'
   "People were eager for information. Many expressed a desire to overcome feelings of helplessness or frustration in dealing with death. They expressed a need for more personal identity and control in the choices they made, similar to the decisions regarding 'natural' childbirth and hospice.
   "One of the serious mistakes I made was to remove John's body before others— his mother and his children—had experienced his death first-hand. Over a year later, for example, when my son Shawn was four years old, he asked, 'But where is my Daddy dead?' The need for involvement of the immediate family was echoed in the various groups with which I spoke. It became clear that all close friends and family should have the opportunity to participate, whenever possible, in ways that lend meaning to each person involved.

"I hope this book will encourage people to become more informed about the choices to be made and less afraid to deal with death. By dealing with the physical aspects of death, emotional needs may be handled effectively as well."
8. Ibid. pp.12–14.

Chapter 27. Honoring the Soul

1. Jack Kornfield, *A Path With Heart: A Guide Through the Perils and Promises of Spiritual Life*, p.34.
2. One of the best books I know for demystifying the process of mindfulness meditation and grounding it in ordinary, everyday experience, is Charlotte Joko Beck's little volume, *Everyday Zen*.
3. John O'Donohue, *Eternal Echoes*, p.94.
4. T. S.Eliot, "Little Gidding" (From *The Four Quartets*).

Chapter 28. Cherishing the Soul

1. John O'Donohue, Anam Cara, pp.173–4. This quote is from the chapter on aging, entitled "Aging: The Beauty of the Inner Harvest."
2. Though an established part of Eastern tradition, in our Western culture, modern literature on dying has only begun to proliferate in recent years, with the work of Elizabeth Kübler-Ross and Stephen Levine. Even so, work on the nuts and bolts of preparing for death is still sparse. An early attempt to fill this gap is Anita Foos-Graber's book *Deathing*. Despite its heavy use of Sanskrit terms, it is a useful book, illustrating theory with an inspirational story of one woman's careful preparation for her own passing.
3. Ram Dass, *Still Here: Embracing Aging Changing and Dying*, p.164–5.
   A spiritual mentor to millions since the 1960s, Ram Dass suffered a stroke in 1997. His speech was affected, and he was confined to a wheelchair. Rather than bemoaning his fate, he embraced it, mining it for even deeper spiritual riches. This book, like its author, is filled with wisdom, insight and humor.

Chapter 29. Kicking the Habits

1. Chellis Glendinning's book title says it all, *My Name Is Chellis And I'm In Recovery From Western Civilization*. "Loving the Earth," she writes, "is a political act." Chellis lives a simple, land-based life in a small community in New Mexico. She has written extensively on the wounding effects of technology and imperialism on the Earth and all its creatures, including ourselves.
2. Joanna Macy, "Working Through Environmental Despair" in T. Roszak, M.E. Gomes, and A.D. Kanner, eds., *Ecopsychology: Restoring the Earth, Healing the Mind*, p.250. Joanna Macy, herself the quintessential elderwoman, has written extensively on this issue of facing up to the pain of the Earth in *World as Lover, World as Self*.
3. From "What's so Good About Feeling Bad?" an interview with Joanna Macy in *New Age Journal*, Jan/Feb, 1991.

Bibliography

ALBERY, N. et al, eds. *The New Natural Death Handbook*. London: The Natural Death Centre, 1997

ALEXANDER, C. et al. *A Pattern Language*. New York: Oxford University Press, 1977

ASSAGIOLI, R. *Psychosynthesis*. New York: Crown, 1979

BECK C J. *Everyday Zen*. San Francisco: Harper, 1989

BELENKY, Mary F. et al. *Women's Ways of Knowing: The Development of Self, Voice, and Mind*. New York: Basic Books, 1986

BERNE, E. *Games People Play: The Psychology Of Human Relationships*. New York: Ballantine, 1996

BIANCHI, E. *Aging as a Spiritual Journey*. New York: Crossroad Publishing, 1982

BLY, R. *The Sibling Society*. Reading, MA: Addison-Wesley, 1996

BOLEN J. S. *Goddesses in Everywoman*. New York: HarperCollins, 1985

———— *Goddesses in Older Women*. New York: HarperCollins, 2001

BOONE, J. Allen. *Kinship With All Life*. New York: Harper & Row, 1954

BRIDGES, W. *Transitions: Making Sense of Life's Changes*. Reading MA: Addison-Wesley, 1980

CARLSON, L. *Caring for the Dead: Your Final Act of Love*. Hinesburg, VT: Upper Access Book Publishers, 1998

CHINEN A. *In the Ever After: Fairy Tales and the Second Half of Life*. Willamette, IL: Chiron, 1989

CHOPRA, D. *Perfect Health: The Complete Mind/Body Guide*. New York: Bantam, 1990

COOPER MARCUS, C. *House as a Mirror of Self: Exploring the Deeper Meaning of Home*. (Berkeley, CA: Conari Press, 1995)

CSIKSZENTMIHALYI, M. *Flow: The Psychology of Optimal Experience*. New York: HarperCollins, 1991

D'ADAMO, Dr. P. et al. *Eat Right for Your Type: The Individualized Diet Solution to Staying Healthy, Living Longer and Achieving Your Ideal Weight*. New York: Putnam, 1997

DAVIS, E, and LEONARD, C. *The Women's Wheel of Life: Thirteen Archetypes of Woman at Her Fullest Power*. New York: Penguin, 1996

276

DIAMOND, J. *The Third Chimpanzee: The Evolution and Future of the Human Animal*. New York: HarperCollins, 1992

DOMINGUEZ, J. and ROBIN, V. *Your Money Or Your Life: Transforming Your Relationship With Money and Achieving Financial Independence*. New York: Penguin, 1993

ERIKSON, E. *Childhood and Society*. New York: W. Norton, 1950

ERIKSON, E. with J. Erikson and H. Kivnick. *Vital Involvement in Old Age*. New York: W.W. Norton, 1986

FERRUCCI, P. *What We May Be: Techniques for Psychological and Spiritual Growth*. (1st ed.) Los Angeles: Tarcher, 1982

FOOS-GRABER, A. *Deathing: An Intelligent Alternative for the Final Moments of Life*. York Beach, ME: Nicolas-Hays Inc., 1989

FOX, W. *Towards a Transpersonal Ecology*. Totnes, Devon (UK): Green Books, 1995

FULGHUM, R. *All I Really Need to Know I Learned in Kindergarten*. New York: Ballantine, 1986

GLENDINNING, C. *My Name Is Chellis and I'm In Recovery From Western Civilization*. Boston MA: Shambhala, 1994

GUTTMAN, D. *Reclaimed Powers: Towards a New Psychology of Men and Women in Later Life*. New York: Basic Books, 1987

HARDING, M. E. *Woman's Mysteries Ancient and Modern*. New York: Harper and Row, 1976

HEILBRUN, C.G. *The Last Gift of Time: Life Beyond Sixty*. New York: Ballantine, 1997

HILLMAN, J. *The Force of Character: And the Lasting Life*. New York: Ballantine, 1999

JACOBS, R. H. *Be an Outrageous Older Woman*. New York: Harper Perennial, 1997

JOHNSON, R. *Owning Your Own Shadow: Understanding the Dark Side of the Psyche*. San Francisco: Harper, 1993

JUNG, C.G. *Collected Works*, edited by Sir H. Read et al., Bollingen Series 20, Princeton, NJ: Princeton University Press, 1954

KINGSTON, K. *Clear Your Clutter With Feng Shui*. New York: Broadway, 1999
———*Creating Sacred Space with Feng Shui*. London: Piatkus, 1996

KOREN, L. *Wabi-Sabi: For Artists, Designers, Poets and Philosophers*. Berkeley, CA: Stone Bridge Press, 1994

KORNFIELD, J.A. *Path With Heart: A Guide Through the Perils and Promises of Spiritual Life*. New York: Bantam, 1993

277

KÜBLER-ROSS, E. *Death: The Final Stage of Growth*. NY: Simon and Schuster, Touchstone 1974

KUSHI, M. (with Alex Jack). *The Book of Macrobiotics: The Universal Way of Health, Happiness, and Peace*. NY: Japan Publications, Inc., 1987

LAO TZU. *Tao Te Ching* . Penguin Classic Edition, 1963

LAWRENCE D. H. *Complete Poems* New York:Viking Penguin, 1994

LEVINE, S. *Who Dies?* New York: Doubleday, 1982

LIEDLOFF, J. *The Continuum Concept: Allowing Human Nature to Work Successfully*. New York: Addison-Wesley, 1977

LUKE, H. *Old Age: Journey into Simplicity*. New York: Parabola, 1987

McCAIN, M. V. *Transformation through Menopause*. New York: Bergin & Garvey, 1991

McDONALD, B. and RICH, C. *Look Me in the Eye: Old Women, Aging, and Ageism*. San Francisco: Spinsters, Ink, 1983

MACY, J. *World as Lover, World as Self*. Berkeley, CA: Parallax Press, 1991

MANKOWITZ, A. *Change of Life: A Psychological Study of Dreams and the Menopause*. Toronto: Inner City Books, 1984

MARTZ, S., ed. *When I am an Old Woman I Shall Wear Purple: An Anthology of Short Stories and Poetry*. Manhattan Beach, CA: Papier-Mache Press, 1987

MOSS R . *The Black Butterfly: An Invitation to Radical Aliveness*. Berkeley, CA: Celestial Arts, 1986

MYSS, C. *Anatomy of the Spirit*. New York: Harmony Books, 1996

NULAND, S. *How We Die: Reflection on Life's Final Chapter*. NY: Alfred A. Knopf, 1994

O'DONOHUE, J. *Anam Cara: A Book of Celtic wisdom*. New York: HarperCollins, 1997
——— *Eternal Echoes: Exploring Our Yearning to Belong*. New York: HarperCollins, 1999

PEARCE, J Chilton. *Evolution's End: Claiming the Potential of Our Intelligence*. San Francisco: Harper, 1995

RAM DASS. *Still Here: Embracing Aging, Changing and Dying*. New York: Riverhead, 2000

RAY, P.H. and S.R. ANDERSON, *The Cultural Creatives: How 50 Million People Are Changing the World* . New York: Harmony Books, 2000

ROSZAK, T. *America the Wise: The Longevity Revolution and the True Wealth of Nations*. New York: Houghton Mifflin, 1998

ROSZAK, T. with M.E. Gomes and A.D. Kanner, eds. *Ecopsychology: Restoring the*

Earth, Healing the Mind. San Francisco: Sierra Club Books, 1995

SCHACHTER-SHALOMI, Z. and R.S. MILLER, *From Age-ing to Sage-ing: A Profound New Vision of Growing Older*. New York: Warner Books, 1995

SCOTT-MAXWELL, F.S. *The Measure of My Days*. New York: Alfred Knopf , 1968

STEINDL-RAST, D. *A Listening Heart*. NY: Crossroad, 1999

SWIMME, B and T. BERRY, *The Universe Story: From the Primordial Flaring Forth to the Ecozoic Era: A Celebration of the Unfolding of the Cosmos*. New York: HarperCollins, 1992

THICH NHAT HANH. *Being Peace*. Berkeley, CA: Parallax Press, 1987

WALKER, B. *The Crone: Woman of Age, Wisdom and Power*. New York: Harper and Row, 1985

————*The Woman's Dictionary of Symbols and Sacred Objects*. New York: Harper and Row, 1988

WOLF, N. *The Beauty Myth: How Images of Beauty are Used Against Women*. New York: William Morrow, 1991

Index